D'Albuquerque's CHILDREN

D'Albuquerque's
CHILDREN

Performing Tradition in Malaysia's Portuguese Settlement

Margaret Sarkissian

The University of Chicago Press
Chicago and London

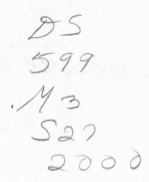

MARGARET SARKISSIAN is associate professor of music at Smith College.

The University of Chicago Press, Chicago 60637
The University of Chicago Press, Ltd., London
© 2000 by The University of Chicago
All rights reserved. Published 2000
Printed in the United States of America
09 08 07 06 05 04 03 02 01 00   5 4 3 2 1

ISBN (cloth): 0-226-73498-6
ISBN (paper): 0-226-73499-4

Library of Congress Cataloging-in-Publication Data

Sarkissian, Margaret.
    D'Albuquerque's children : performing tradition in Malaysia's Portuguese settlement /
Margaret Sarkissian.
        p.   cm. — (Chicago studies in ethnomusicology)
    Includes bibliographical references (p.   ) and index.
    ISBN 0-226-73498-6 (cloth) — ISBN 0-226-73499-4 (pbk.)
    1. Portuguese—Malaysia—Malacca (Malacca)   2. Performing arts—Malaysia—
Malacca (Malacca)   I. Title.   II. Series.
DS599.M3 S27   2000
959.5'1004691—dc21

00-008517

For Uncle Noel, Papa Joe, and my godson, Jeremy

Contents

Illustrations

Tables

I would like to express my eternal gratitude to the people of the Portuguese Settlement in Malacca. This is their story, and without their collective generosity and patience, I would not have been able to write it. It is not easy to pick out a few names for special thanks, but I should mention Emmanuel Bosco "Joe" Lazaroo, Noel Felix, Cypriano Francis "Sub" de Costa, and Gerard de Costa in particular. Thanks are also due (alphabetically) to Basil Bournaparte, the late Georgie de Costa, Josephine de Costa, Patrick, Fidelis, and Sebastian de Silva, Gerard Fernandis, Laura Martinez, Norman de Mello, George Bosco Lazaroo, the late Louis Lazaroo, Oliver Lazaroo, Aloysius Sta. Maria, Bertie Sta. Maria, Tony and Joseph Sta. Maria, the late Freddie Scully, Michael Singho, Stephen Theseira, Michael Young, and all the musicians and dancers of Tropa de Malaca and Rancho Folclorico San Pedro. I am extremely grateful to Anne and Gerard de Costa, Carrieanne, Jeremy, and the entire extended de Mello and de Costa families (not forgetting Yong Kok Chong) for allowing me to become part of the family. I am also grateful to Syed Salleh, Ramah Arshad, and family and to Sukhjit Singh and family for opening their homes to me whenever I needed to stay in Kuala Lumpur.

I owe an enormous amount to my teachers, especially to Bruno Nettl, Edward M. Bruner, Charles Capwell, and David Stigberg for opening up a whole new world of thoughts and ideas. I would like to thank Clark Cunningham in particular who, in addition to shepherding me through the traumas of the original dissertation, has remained a mentor, advisor, and valued friend as the research continued and the study grew into a book. These are debts that can never be repaid directly: instead, I hope I can grow to inspire my students as profoundly as you have all inspired me.

I greatly appreciate the kindness of colleagues who not only read and commented on portions of this book but also have remained my friends: Alan Baxter, Rodger Blum, Clark Cunningham, Sue Darlington, John Hellweg, K. David Jackson, Donald Joralemon, Frederick Lau, Marian Macdonald, Robert C. Provine, Alyn Shipton, Ruth Solie, William Seigh, and Larry Witzleben. It is a better work for your help; the remaining infelicities are purely my own. I am also grateful to other friends who read and commented on earlier versions of this project, in particular Mohd Anis Md Nor, Mars Cavers, Patricia Matusky, Judy McCulloh, Marc Perlman, Wayne Stier, Tan Sooi Beng, and M. Veera Pandiyan, to José Moças for producing the CD *Kantiga di Padri să Chang,* to Susana Sardo for Portuguese translations for the CD, to Alec McLane for preparing the musical examples, and to Jane Domier for drawing the maps. I would like to thank T. David Brent for a decade of encouragement, the anonymous University of Chicago Press readers who gave me so much food for thought, and Richard Allen, copyeditor and fellow accordionist.

I gratefully acknowledge all the funding I have received over the past decade to make this extended study of the Portuguese Settlement possible. The original dissertation research, conducted over a period of fifteen months (1990–91), was made possible by grants from the Theodore Presser Foundation, the Royal Anthropological Institute of Great Britain and Ireland, and the Graduate College of the University of Illinois at Urbana-Champaign. In addition, I would like to thank the Malaysian government's Socio-Economic Research Unit and the Universiti Sains Malaysia's Pusat Seni (Arts Center) for arranging my research permit and providing the necessary academic affiliation. Subsequent shorter trips in 1994, 1996, and 1998 were funded by summer research grants from Smith College, and course release time was provided by a Harvey Picker fellowship.

My deepest appreciation is reserved for my parents, Arshak and Edwina, my sister Jenny, and for the special friends who have kept me going through the years: Anis, John Hellweg, Fred Lau, my *adik* Lee Tong Soon, Marc Perlman, Rob Provine, Nancy Schertler, Ruth Solie, and Yosihiko Tokumaru. Rodger Blum and William Seigh co-existed graciously with this book throughout the five years that we shared a home. No one could have a better group of cheerleaders.

Language

The residents of the Portuguese Settlement are, to varying degrees, trilingual. Most speak a mixture of the local Portuguese creole (called Kristang), English, and Malay. Older residents of lower socioeconomic status tend to be Kristang dominant in daily life; middle-aged residents and those of middle- to higher socioeconomic status tend to be English dominant; young children who attend government schools are more fluent in Malay than are their parents and grandparents. Kristang, while used frequently in the home, is an oral language; it is rarely written down. I have thus chosen to follow the Australian linguist Alan Baxter's (1987, 1988) orthography, which reflects the close connection between Kristang and Bahasa Malaysia, rather than attempting any kind of quasi-Portuguese spelling as preferred by the few Settlement residents who write in Kristang.

Song texts originally set in Kristang are easily transcribed and translated into English. Texts originally set in Portuguese, however, present complex challenges for the translator. Since these songs have been transmitted orally, singers often approximate sounds or even substitute Kristang words or phrases. In these cases, I have tried to transcribe the words exactly as they are sung (following Baxter's orthography, where possible), but because coherent translation is often impossible, Portuguese versions have been used for English translations. It is, of course, probably fair to assume that my approximation of the singer's approximated sounds adds a further layer of incoherence to the song text.

Recordings

Most of the musical items discussed in this book can be found on the compact disc, *Kantiga di Padri să Chang: Malaca* (Tradisom VS 05). This compact disc is available for purchase from Tradisom, Editora Discografica, I.D.A, Apartado 69, 4730 Vila Verde, Portugal. It may also be ordered through Tradisom's web site, which is located at http://www.tradisom.pt.

INTRODUCTION

This book is about the ways music, identity, tradition, and tourism interact in a rather unusual village in Malaysia. The village is located halfway between Kuala Lumpur and Singapore, just outside the city of Malacca (see map 1). It was created in the mid-1920s at the tail end of the British colonial period as a kind of reservation for a people thought to be on the verge of cultural extinction. The only such village in Malaysia, its residents make it even more distinct. Of mixed European and Asian descent, they are a living reminder of a colonial past. Despite bearing a variety of Portuguese, Dutch, and British family names, they call themselves Malaysian-Portuguese, Luso-Malays, or simply Portuguese descendants, speak a Portuguese creole which they call Kristang, and practice the Roman Catholic faith. The village has thus become known as the Portuguese Settlement, or Kampung Portugis in Malay.

While this book is a case study at heart, an exploration of the way traditions are invented and reinvented through performance in one particular community, it is also a paradigmatic tale of postmodernism. On the one hand, the village and its residents have straddled the transition between colonial and postcolonial worlds and navigated the ups and downs of life in post-independence Malaysia with a certain amount of ingenuity and, at times, panache. Though the residents form a tiny fraction of the two percent of the Malaysian population identified in the official statistics as "Other" (i.e., not Malay, Chinese, or Indian) and have little in the way of political or economic capital, they have imaginatively made the most of what they have—a quaint living space and an "exotic" culture, exotic by virtue of being "European" in the middle of Asia—to put themselves on the map nationally and even, in certain circles, internationally. On the other hand, they also straddle a vast network of communities of Portuguese descent stretching from Goa and Sri Lanka to Macau. These communities have much in common in terms of social, political, and cultural

Map 1
Malacca town and environs.

MALACCA TOWN AND ENVIRONS

a. St. Peter's Church
b. St. Francis Xavier's Church
c. Christ Church and Clock Tower
d. Stadthuys
e. St. Paul's Church (ruin)
f. Santiago Gate
g. Independence Memorial Museum (formerly Malacca Club)
h. St. Francis Institute (boys' school)
i. Assumption Chapel
j. St. John's Fort (ruin)

TENGKERA (Tranquerah)
to Port Dickson

Gajah Berang

to Kuala Lumpur

to Bukit Pinggir

BUKIT PIATU

to Bukit Baru

Bukit Serindit

SEMABOK

BUKIT CHINA

St. John's Hill

UJONG PASIR

to Singapore

Bandar Hilir

Praya Lane

Garden City

(Malacca Raya)

Reclaimed Land

Reclaimed Land

Straits of Malacca

Portuguese Settlement

Chew Loy "hamlet"

PADANG TEMU

0   1/4   1/2
Mile

PENINSULAR MALAYSIA

Penang

Kuala Lumpur

Kuantan

Malacca

SINGAPORE

Straits of Malacca

0   100
Miles

Dornier

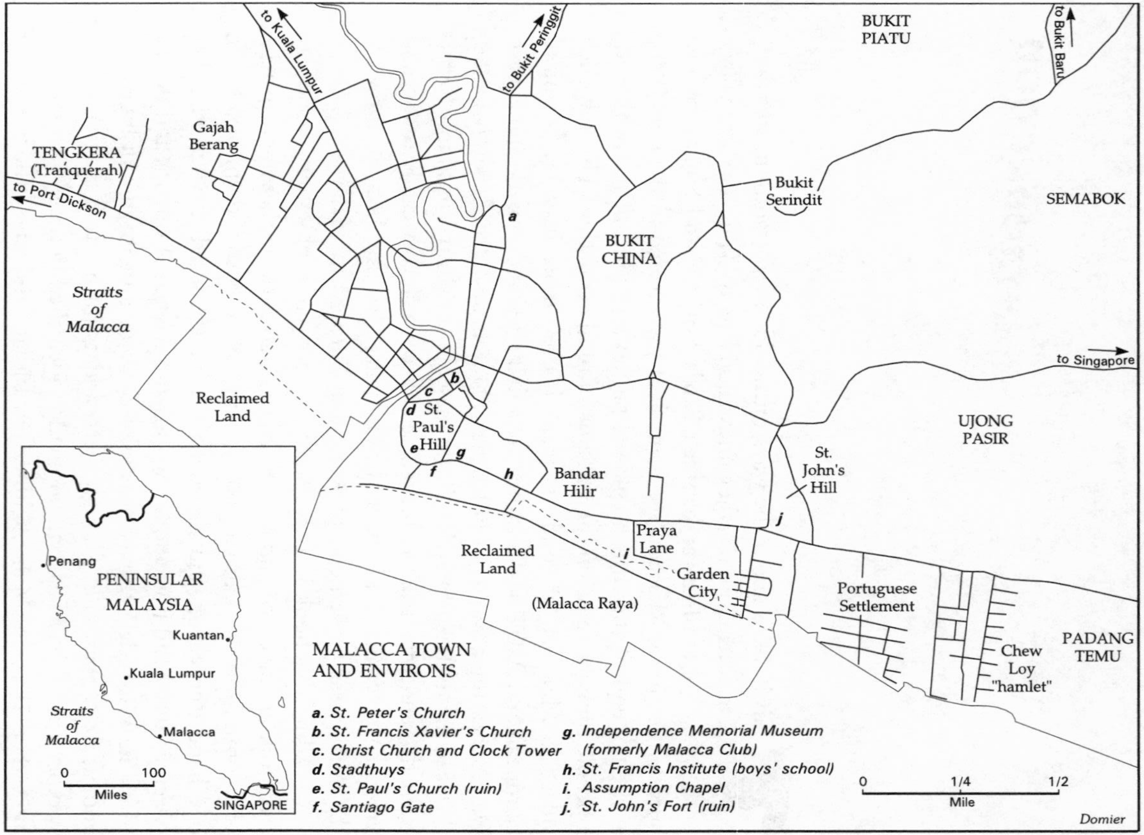

organization, as is now becoming apparent through comparative collections such as Tradisom's series of twelve compact discs, *a viagem dos sons/ the journey of sounds.*

• • •

I went to the Portuguese Settlement in 1990 to do fieldwork for a doctoral dissertation (Sarkissian 1993). Having completed a master's thesis that examined the ways music marked social and political divisions in the Armenian immigrant community of Toronto (Sarkissian 1987), I was particularly interested in exploring similar issues among minorities in a postcolonial context. I had also recently read Hobsbawm and Ranger's 1983 collection *The Invention of Tradition,* and was curious about the role "tradition" played in defining one's place in a new nation. Picking a nation was easy: Malaysia combined my love of Southeast Asia (and its foods), which had begun with a summer in Indonesia during my final year of high school, with my interest in multicultural societies. In fact, immediately before starting graduate school in 1984 I spent a summer in Malaysia, testing the waters to see if I really did want to become an ethnomusicologist.

I had heard about the Portuguese Settlement during that preliminary visit, but finally settled on it as a dissertation topic after two accidents in the University of Illinois library and one extraordinary piece of good luck. The first accident occurred when, looking for something else in the main library, I ran across a slim book called *My People, My Country* by a man called Bernard Sta. Maria (1982). Despite my gnawing fear of being crushed by the motorized stacks, I sat down on the floor and read the book from cover to cover, captivated by the tale he told of Malacca's Portuguese community from its glorious sixteenth-century past to its modest twentieth-century present. Bernard wrote passionately about preserving his culture and reviving lapsed traditions, including festivals, music, and dance. Wondering whether Bernard's "revived" traditions might in fact be newly "invented" traditions, it dawned on me that this village might be a good place to explore further the interactions between music, identity, and tradition. One of my greatest regrets is that I never had the opportunity to meet or interview Bernard Sta. Maria. Though I came to know his brothers Tony and Joseph well, Bernard died two and a half years before I found his book on the library shelf.

The second accident occurred some months later in the mustiest nether regions of the newspaper library as I was looking through back issues of one of Malaysia's English-language newspapers, the *New Straits Times*. The enormous pile of papers on the desk in front of me toppled over and spilled onto the floor. Surveying the mess, I noticed something I had missed the first time around: a colorful picture of musicians and dancers wearing costumes that looked distinctly Iberian. The picture turned out to be part of a feature on the traditional music of the Portuguese Settlement as performed by Joe Lazaroo and his cultural troupe, Rancho Folclorico San Pedro. I remembered Bernard's book and wondered again about the incongruity between the costumes, which looked so familiarly Portuguese, and the faces, which looked distinctly Malay. I am not sure why—perhaps because it was cold and February in Illinois—but I thought it might be worth a stamp to write and ask Joe Lazaroo about his music. I addressed my letter to "Joe Lazaroo, Portuguese Settlement, Malacca, Malaysia" and soon forgot about it. In early June, literally as I was leaving the music school to fly to Malaysia, the receptionist ran after me waving a letter that had just arrived with a Malaysian stamp. I put the letter in my jacket pocket and was half way to O'Hare airport before I looked at it and discovered, to my great surprise, that it was from Joe Lazaroo and contained detailed instructions on how to get from Kuala Lumpur to Malacca and the Portuguese Settlement. Having known Joe Lazaroo for more than a decade now, I am amazed not that my letter found its way to the right Joe Lazaroo, nor that I received his answer as I was on my way to the airport. The extraordinary piece of good luck was that Joe actually replied to my inquiry. As he is fond of telling everyone, he never answers his mail.

As anyone who does fieldwork knows (but seldom publicly admits), much of one's success is dependent on a serendipitous conjunction of persons, time, and place. In this case, everything seemed to point to the Portuguese Settlement as an auspicious location for my particular combination of interests. And better yet, it promised to be a manageable, contained topic. As James Clifford (1997, 21) has observed, "Villages, inhabited by natives, are bounded sites particularly suitable for intensive visiting by anthropologists. They have long served as habitable, mappable centers for the community and, by extension, the culture." Of course, convenient as such a bounded site may be, there is another side to working in small villages: the smaller the site, the more intense the visit, the deeper the roots one puts down. After fifteen months of life in the Portuguese Settlement (from June 1990 to August 1991), I was in Clifford's terms a "homebody abroad" (22).

The importance residents of the Settlement attached to relationships was impressed on me early in my stay by Bernard Sta. Maria's brother, Tony. One day while we were sitting at Jenny's coffee shop, he said (with a little bitterness in his voice), "You know, you *Ropiano*s [Kristang: 'Europeans'] come here to study us and our ways. We take you as our daughter or our sister and you become part of our lives. Then you go back to your country and we don't see you some more." Since Joe Lazaroo is by no means unusual in his reluctance to answer mail, physically going back has seemed the least I could do to show that I cared beyond the limits of a dissertation. In so doing, I have acquired a second life, an adopted family, and an imp of a godson. Now, like all good Settlement residents who work "outstation," I do my best to *balik kampung* (Malay: "return home") for the annual Festa di San Pedro, the festival of Saint Peter, the patron saint of the Settlement. In the summers of 1992, 1994, 1996, and 1998, I returned for periods of six to ten weeks; in 1997 and 1999 I managed only fleeting week-long visits en route to other work in Japan.

At the outset, I intended to produce the kind of musical ethnography that has abounded in my discipline, ethnomusicology. To that end, I adopted the "participant observer" approach and started to learn about music by learning to play it. Since my own instrument, the trumpet, was not part of the Settlement soundscape, I decided to take up something that was—the accordion. This was probably my smartest single fieldwork move because, despite having no prior experience, I was immediately in great demand. Though competent guitarists were a dime a dozen in the Portuguese Settlement, there was only one other accordionist and he only played sporadically for one group. Within three months of my arrival, I had figured out how to play it (after a fashion), learned most of the regular repertoire (thanks to the dedicated and generous assistance of "Sub" de Costa), and without ever consciously having made the decision to play in public, was performing regularly with two different groups, Rancho Folclorico San Pedro and Tropa de Malaca.[1]

I quickly realized that in addition to my three original research topics—music, identity, and tradition—I would have to take into account a fourth: tourism. I could not escape the fact that I was now living in the middle of one of Malacca's prime tourist attractions and that music and dance were a crucial part of the package. In fact, music and dance have become so closely associated with the Portuguese Settlement that as far as a large portion of the Malaysian general public is concerned, the Settlement *is* a village of musicians and dancers dressed in Portuguese costume.[2] Speaking of the Portuguese Mechanics (a similar mixed-race community in Sri Lanka) during the British colonial period, McGilvray (1982, 245) notes: "They were recognized to have a certain flair for music, dancing, revelry, and bright costumes, although these were scarcely seen as redeeming virtues." This ambivalent verging on negative association between music, dance, and Portuguese heredity is a colonial-period stereotype that still exerts a powerful fascination in postcolonial Malaysia. The identification between music, dance, costume, and "authentic" Portuguese Eurasian identity is now so strong that—like the Aborigines and Navajo described by Thomas (1994, 30) who speak English and wear western clothes—those who do not conform to expectations do not count as real "natives." This, of course, raises fascinating questions about authenticity, an issue that permeates much of this book. Rather than seeing authenticity as part of a black and white dichotomy (authentic/inauthentic), I am inclined to agree with Bruner (1994, 408), who suggests that it should be viewed instead "as a struggle, a social process, in which competing interests argue for their own interpretation of history." By identifying four meanings of authenticity—based on verisimilitude (is it credible and convincing?), genuineness (is it an immaculate simulation?), originality (is it the "real thing"?), and authority (is it duly certified?)—Bruner (400–401) has established a model that encourages a more fruitful exploration of the issues surrounding the construction of authenticity, the nature of the authority that legitimizes it, and the way both are in a constant process of being invented and reinvented.

Closer examination of the performing tradition showed that—like Nigerian *jùjú* as described by The Honourable Joshua Olufemi—it was, in fact, "a very modern tradition" (Waterman 1990, 378). Performed by a limited number of musicians and dancers, including teenagers equally skilled in the latest hip-hop moves, it is a "tradition" designed specifically to display the past—or, more accurately, an imagined past—to outsiders, including transient tourists and visiting dignitaries. At the same time, an older style of vocal performance that I (wearing my ethnomusicologist's hat) might call "traditional music" has been virtually abandoned, considered by its practitioners to be too hybrid and not traditional enough. Delving deeper into the musical world of the Settlement led to explorations of traditions that are invented and reinvented through performance, ways a community represents itself and is represented by others, and the constant dialogic interaction between real and fictive constructions of self and community.

The more I learned about the Portuguese Settlement and its residents over the years, the more I came to realize that the social, cultural, and historical web in which they are embedded was far more intricate than I had suggested in my original dissertation. When I started to write this book, writing ethnography became both a form of detective work and an exercise in writing history—history as imagined as well as history that actually happened, for "no ethnography can ever hope to penetrate beyond the surface planes of everyday life, to plumb its invisible forms, unless it is informed by the historical imagination—the imagination, that is, of both those who make history and those who write [and tell] it" (Comaroff and Comaroff 1992, xi).[3] At the heart of the web stands a singular community: a people of acknowledged mixed race, part European, part Asian, who live in a resettlement village in the middle of Southeast Asia, a human example of "the functioning of colonial power as a form of transaction and translation between incommensurable cultures and positions" (Prakash 1995, 3). Understanding the Settlement as it was when founded in the mid-1920s—a nostalgic attempt to salvage an idealized precolonial (or at least, pre-British colonial) community on the verge of "destruction" (see Thomas 1994, 15)—is quite different from understanding the Settlement in its contemporary postcolonial context—a vestige of history in which make-believe Europeans are contained and displayed. In this regard, I owe much to recent work in anthropology and cultural studies, particularly those works that attempt to recuperate colonial history and reconsider postcolonial rewritings of the historical record (see, e.g., Breckenridge and van der Veer 1993; Luhrmann 1996; Prakash 1995; Thomas 1994; and Young 1995).

Perhaps influenced by the countless tourists I saw watching this world through camera viewfinders and certainly encouraged by the ways James Clifford has juxtaposed "experiments in travel writing and poetic collage" (1997, 12) with more conventional scholarly discourse, I have tried to capture some of the ambience of the experience. To this end, the book is suffused with vignettes drawn from my field notes and embellished with what Gage Averill has called "head notes" or memories (1997, xi). These vignettes inevitably juxtapose contrasting images of the early modern and the postmodern, the colonial and the postcolonial. In addition to providing starting points for the ensuing discussions, the images form a cinematographic sequence, zooming from a wide-angled picture-postcard view of the Settlement as a tourist sight/site to a close-up behind-the-scenes look at a single performance. Progressing literally from "front stage" to "back stage" (MacCannell 1976), the sequence also mirrors my own journey as a fieldworker. At the outset, I saw the Settlement with the eyes of a tourist; today I not only see the Settlement with different eyes, but also in my capacity as performer, friend, advocate, and godmother, have become part of the picture.

• • •

June 1990 Zorro's position could hardly have been more desperate when we were suddenly catapulted from a Hollywood rerun into a commercial break. Instead of a jaunty jingle extolling the virtues of yet another product guaranteed to make our lives easier, mysterious music began to emanate from a swirling gray mist. Slowly a nebulous image formed: as calm gray sea melted into cold gray sky, a ghostly apparition floated eerily toward us through thinning fog. As the mist cleared, the shadows coalesced into a ship, a huge wooden ship, European in style, with white canvas sails hanging wraith-like from proud yardarms. Though the image remained artistically blurred, the reference was crystal clear to everyone sitting around the flickering television set: the year was 1511 and we were witnessing Afonso de Albuquerque's flagship, the *Flor de la Mar,* sail silently into the fabled port of Malacca. An instant later, magically transported to the present, we were bombarded by a kaleidoscopic array of current attractions flashing above a single command—"Visit Malacca, Malaysia's Historic City"—while disembodied voices sang sweetly, assuring us that in "Malaysia . . . there's so much more you can . . . discover." It was at this point that my new acquaintances lost interest. After all, why should they visit Malacca, when they live in the middle of one of the attractions just seen on the screen? As I continued to mull over the issues raised by the commercial, everyone else's attention had refocused on something far more exciting—a trailer for the next show, *MacGyver.*

• • •

This television commercial was part of a series (each one of which advertised the attractions of a different state) produced by the Malaysian Tourist Development Corporation during Visit Malaysia Year 1990. This particular commercial focused on Malaysia's third smallest state, Malacca. With little in the way of natural resources (no clean sandy beaches, exotic fauna, or spectacular scenery), the state government has constructed a highly successful tourist industry around Malacca's twin assets: history and heritage. According to legend, the town was founded in about 1400 by the Palembang-born prince, Parameswara. As the story goes, while out hunting one day, Parameswara watched his dogs chase a small mousedeer up a hill.[4] When the mousedeer reached the summit, it turned to face its pursuers. The dogs were so startled by the mousedeer's unexpected bravery that they tumbled down the hill and into the river. Parameswara chose this hill, the place where the weak stood up to the strong, as the site for a new settlement. Since then, the city has remained at the heart of Malaysia's history. Conquered in turn by the Portuguese (1511), the Dutch (1647), and the British (1824) and occupied during World War II by the Japanese, it was the place where in 1956 Tunku Abdul Rahman (soon to become Malaysia's first prime minister) emulated the mousedeer and announced the nation's forthcoming independence. Malacca's cultural heritage is equally rich. Because of its early significance as an international entrepôt, the city attracted traders from all over the world. Many of these merchants made cosmopolitan Malacca their home, some took local wives, and gradually new communities evolved. Today, in addition to the three major races of Malaysia (Malay, Chinese, and Indian), there are other long-standing minorities who call Malacca their home: the Baba-Nonyas (Straits-born Chinese or *Peranakans* in Malay), the Chitty Melaka (Straits-born Indians), and the Portuguese Eurasians.[5]

As the commercial demonstrates, a vaguely romanticized Portuguese past is a crucial theme in the state government's marketing of the city as "Historical Malacca: The Place Where It All Began." Not content with monuments that are "the real thing" in Bruner's taxonomy (like the Santiago Gate, the only surviving part of Albuquerque's fortress), the state government has manufactured and "duly certified" a number of new memorials, including a replica of Albuquerque's *Flor de la Mar*. Today, when you walk through Malacca's designated "historical area," you cannot miss the treasure "ship," which—though it looks like a ship-shape sea-going vessel—is actually a ship-shaped air-conditioned museum moored in concrete alongside the Malacca River. But monuments, whether real or invented, serve to construct memory and structure history (Wu Hung 1995, 4). Despite their aura and patina of age, they are little more than a series of static photo opportunities. To enhance Malacca's position as Malaysia's premier destination for cultural tourism, image makers have added living color by co-opting the Portuguese Settlement and its residents.

In Historical Malacca the Portuguese Settlement is both a monument/attraction tourists visit to view "natives" going about their daily business (much as they might look at exotic animals in a game park) and a venue where they go to eat, drink, and be entertained by musicians and dancers in Portuguese dress. It is hardly surprising, then, that an extraordinarily complex relationship has developed between the Settlement, on the one hand, as a designated historical sight/site and, on the other, as a real-life living space. At its most glamorous, the Settlement-as-historical-monument is filled with shadows of the past that mingle with shadows of imagined or wished-for pasts, and which in turn affect our understanding of the everyday Settlement-as-housing-estate. Newspapers, guidebooks, and documentaries locate the Settlement anywhere between a reconstructed pioneer village and a vestigial slice of living history, most often portraying it as a poor fishing village filled with worthy folk who struggle heroically against the odds to maintain their age-old customs, language, and traditions. This is what tourists *expect* to see and—strangely enough—it is what many actually *do* see: by measuring reality against a preconceived image it is possible to selectively edit out the bits that do not fit. In this way one can overlook the high school, standing squarely since 1949 in the middle of the Settlement, while accepting the Portuguese Square—constructed (on the opposite side of the concrete parking lot) by the government in 1985—as a piece of old Portugal. Preconceived images of this sort are crucial to the tourist imagination. As tourists, how many of us have traveled with guidebooks open, measuring the actual sight we see against the written or photographed account, checking it off the list as we go? As Edward Bruner (1995, 233) notes, "The touristic mode of experiencing is primarily visual, and to have been there, to have 'seen' it, only requires presence. The tourist 'sees' enough of the . . . ritual to confirm his prior images derived from the media, from brochures and from *National Geographic*." Significantly, as we shall see, this shadowy world exists not only in the minds of tourists and government publicity officers; it is also slowly taking root in the minds of Settlement residents themselves.

At the same time, one cannot avoid the fact that the Settlement is also a functioning living space. Despite what the tour guides would have us believe, it does not date back to 1511 but was founded and developed as a reservation during the last years of British rule. Today, of course, it is another world. At its most prosaic, it is a world rooted in late-twentieth-century transglobal culture. As we glimpsed above, residents watch *Zorro* and *MacGyver,* rent movies, and go into debt to possess cars; their children listen to the latest Malaysian or international pop phenomena, wear the sort of clothes one might see in an American inner city, and eat or work at McDonald's. Although there is still a good deal of conspicuous poverty, many families are tearing down their patchwork wooden houses, replacing them with new stone buildings, and gradually filling them with all the conveniences of modern life—refrigerators, washing machines, TVs, VCRs, DVDs, stereos, and even karaoke sets. Residents pass between these two worlds—the Settlement-as-historical-monument and the Settlement-as-housing-estate—with consummate ease. Many go about their daily business, oblivious to the tour buses that rumble past their homes; tourists are part of the scenery—as faceless to them as they, in their everyday clothes, are to the tourists. But others come home from work or school, put on Portuguese costumes and dancing shoes, pick up guitars, and head for the bright lights of the stage. For the stage is the meeting ground, the place where the two worlds collide.

Herein lies the rub: the music, dance, and costumes that have come to represent the Portuguese Settlement exist solely on stage within the confines of the cultural show; they are not used by residents for their own purposes (e.g., at community events such as festivals, weddings, dances, etc.). This crucial detail invites us to reexamine the cultural show not as a genre maligned by "serious" scholars (who often dismiss such shows as "inauthentic," "superficial," or "just for tourists") but as a contemporary "text" to be interpreted.[6] In so doing, we discover a wealth of what Renato Rosaldo (1989, 208) has called "sites of creative cultural production." These creative spaces, which Bruner (1996, 159) suggests exist in a "touristic borderzone," provide opportunities "for the invention of culture on a massive scale." Viewed in this light, the cultural show becomes a lively forum, a government-sanctioned space in which ethnic difference is tolerated, even encouraged, and where the primary function is communication between worlds (Sarkissian 1997, 1998a). At the same time, it is a "site of struggle" (Clifford 1997, 212) in which people display themselves or are displayed. Stories people choose to tell about themselves compete with myths created (by them or by others) in order to fulfill audience expectations. In this fertile borderzone, diverse and often competing messages co-exist and speak simultaneously to different audiences. Just what these voices choose to say and/or what actors and consumers choose to hear are factors subject to constant negotiation, revision, and (re)interpretation.

This dynamic state is nowhere more complex and volatile than in rapidly developing postcolonial nations like Malaysia (see Nash 1989, 21–60). As fast as governments try to forge national unity, to link unknown peoples together in "imagined communities" (Anderson 1983), discrete ethnic groups resist, subtly or overtly, by marking their individual difference. The expression of ethnic difference, whether "a top-down imposition from the powerful, or a grass-roots response to humiliations and frustrations," is often encouraged by governments, because it is a powerful diversion, a way of focusing attention away from the more pressing issues, such as class difference (Kipp 1996, 71). In such situations, the cultural show—already a safe, government-sanctioned space—becomes a wider public forum that transcends the touristic borderzone to become a national battlefield where meaning is contested and identity negotiated. Tension exists between official government-sponsored professional troupes that represent "the nation" (in terms of membership as well as product) and local community troupes that represent specific minority interests. Government troupes perform varied and eclectic "traditional" material presented as representative of all the nation's peoples, to create an image of multiethnic tolerance and national harmony (see Kirshenblatt-Gimblett 1998, 64–65; Sarkissian 1998a). This image, seemingly directed toward outsiders (visiting dignitaries and businessmen as well as tourists), generates international recognition, investment, and valuable foreign exchange. But—perhaps more insidiously—the message is also directed by the government toward insiders, presenting happy multicultural coexistence (which may be little more than a glittering illusion) as established reality.

The position of grassroots cultural troupes (like those found in the Portuguese Settlement) is much more complicated. Though their formation is often encouraged by the government, local desire to display difference implicitly critiques government attempts to create national unity.[7] Such troupes tread a fine line between co-option, subversion, and plain pragmatism. Performing distinct "traditional" material of their own, they function as social safety valves; by this means governments, in effect, contain minorities by giving them the illusion of freedom of expression. Overt ethnic diversity, discouraged in more sensitive domains (such as religion), "is valued, honoured, even apotheosized, but only as long as it remains at the level of display, not belief, performance, not enactment" (Acciaioli 1985, 161). In other words, from the government perspective, ethnic diversity is acceptable when confined to the rigidly defined, nonthreatening, transient domain of performance. Conscious or not of the extent to which they are being co-opted, ethnic minorities manipulate the situation just as deftly, either subverting the government's message under its very nose or superficially complying for material advantage. From the local perspective, cultural shows can be either "stolen opportunities," fleeting chances to circulate knowledge privately and display difference publicly with impunity (Aragon 1996, 435), or a pragmatic way of enhancing the community's position in a rapidly changing world.

In performances given by government-sponsored professional troupes or by local troupes of different ethnic backgrounds who happen to be sharing the same stage, the cultural show has become the performing equivalent of theme parks such as Taman Mini "Indonesia Indah" ("Beautiful Indonesia"-in-Miniature) or the Malaysian version, Mini Malaysia. Just as each of Indonesia's twenty-six provinces is represented at Taman Mini by a single house built in an ahistoric "genuine customary architectural style" (Pemberton 1994, 152), so each item on a cultural show program is a stereotypical distillation representing the music and dance of a particular region or ethnic group. Superficially aimed at tourists, such productions are equally (if not more) powerful for urban residents who have little practical experience of life outside the modern metropolis. In their "miniaturized clarity," Taman Mini's houses become substitutes for "home" in the mind of urban individuals as far from home mentally as they are geographically (Pemberton 1994, 157–59); the neatly packaged songs and dances of the cultural show become substitutes for "tradition" in the minds of urban Malaysians more familiar with westernized popular music than with anything that might be called traditional performing arts. Gradually (as Picard [1990, 1996] and Bruner [1995] have both demonstrated in Bali), tourist performances may be reabsorbed into the host culture to the point that they are accepted by local audiences as traditional. This process is further complicated in the case of the Portuguese Settlement: the stereotypical distillation that has come to represent the Settlement to the outside world and that is gradually becoming accepted by residents as part of their own tradition is derived not from indigenous Settlement traditions linking the contemporary community to its sixteenth-century heritage but from twentieth-century Portuguese importations.

At the same time, older indigenous Settlement traditions are dying out because they are considered too hybrid and not "traditional" enough. Although this move from hybrid to ethnically distinct genres might appear to reverse the more common pattern of change, it connects the Portuguese Settlement to a broader national movement in the arts away from colonial cosmopolitanism toward postcolonial segregation. Government attempts to forge a unifying national culture have resulted in a growing tendency toward ethnic segregation, marked in the arts as well as in politics and other aspects of daily life. For example, the theatrical genre *bangsawan* is described today as "traditional Malay theater" (Ramah Bujang 1975), but, as Tan Sooi Beng has carefully demonstrated, such a definition is essentially a modern interpretation grounded in a highly politicized context.

During the colonial period *bangsawan* was, in fact, a commercially successful multiethnic form of urban popular theater performed by Malays, Eurasians, Chinese, Indians, Filipinos, and Arabs who lived, worked, and traveled together (Tan 1989a, 250; see also Tan 1989b). Constantly adapting to changing audience tastes and exploiting the latest vaudeville crazes, *bangsawan* provided a forum for the interaction of foreign and local musics:

> [With a repertoire] stocked with Western, Malay, Indian, Chinese, Javanese, Spanish, Egyptian, Turkish and other foreign stories, dances, and songs [*bangsawan* was] "modern," "up-to-date," "heterogenetic," and "innovative," . . . it was the popular non-European commercial urban theater for different ethnic groups living all over Malaya. (Tan 1989a, 255–56; see also Tan 1993)

As the Independence movement gained momentum during the 1940s and 1950s, Malay historical tales became increasingly popular as subject matter for *bangsawan* performances. It was not until the 1970s that the government, faced with the task of redefining national identity in the wake of post-election ethnically based riots, actively appropriated the genre and began to reformulate it based on a core of supposedly "traditional" Malay cultural values (Tan 1989a, 253). Hybrid and multicultural elements—non-Malay plots, songs, instruments, and performers—were dropped as *bangsawan* was "reshaped, Malayized and institutionalized for new national purposes" (Tan 1989b, 9). In modern "traditional" *bangsawan,* improvisation has given way to fixed scripts; popular songs have been replaced with newly composed "Malay" songs; and the comic interludes known as "extra turns" have been eliminated altogether (Ramah Bujang 1992, 8–9). In effect, government intervention has transformed *bangsawan* from popular to "traditional" theater, alienating the original multicultural urban audience along the way. *Bangsawan* may have been elevated to the status of high art, but it now appeals only to a small, educated city audience. As Tan concludes, shows have become

> too "fixed" and "formal." Although the sets and costumes were designed for historical detail and exhibited courtly extravagance, and rituals of the Malay court were observed in great detail, the Ministry of Culture's *bangsawan* did not cater to the audience's tastes. As Utih [a local theater critic] emphasizes, the "soul of *bangsawan* was missing." (Tan 1989a, 256)

A similar transformation occurred in the case of *zapin melayu,* a village folk dance from Johor, the southernmost state in the peninsula

(Mohd Anis Md Nor 1993). Derived from *zapin arab,* *zapin melayu* still retains a strong Islamic flavor; Arabic rhythms are played on a hand-held frame drum, and melodies are played on the *gambus,* the Malay term for the Arabic lute, *'ūd* (Mohd Anis Md Nor 1990, 30). In the prewar era, *zapin melayu* (then an informal line dance performed only by men) was popular fare at wedding celebrations, where it served simultaneously as secular entertainment and religious celebration (ibid., 39–42). Made popular by *bangsawan* performers and the growing Malay film industry, *zapin melayu* became nationally known during the 1940s and 1950s. Perhaps because of its Islamic associations, the dance was deemed suitable for appropriation by the government as it attempted to construct a national culture in the 1970s. Reformulated and refined, the national *zapin* is no longer a spontaneous, participatory dance. Instead, it has become an elaborate choreographed production performed most visibly by massed ranks of schoolchildren (of both sexes) in football stadiums for state events. In the process, the national *zapin*—like *bangsawan*—has lost much of its characteristic flexibility and its wide range of improvisational capabilities (ibid., 244). Unlike *bangsawan,* however, the village *zapin melayu* continues to be performed by an aging population in the Johor region. Furthermore, with the encouragement of Prof. Anis and the Johor state government, *zapin melayu* has been reintroduced on a large scale to Johor's younger generation.

Bangsawan and *zapin* are just two examples of genres "Malayized" as a result of the government's attempt to invent a "national culture." In both cases, institutionalization resulted in increased rigidity as invented traditions—essentially fixed showpieces categorized as "Malaysian culture"—were presented in novel contexts to a newly created national audience. But what about the former multiethnic dimension? Presenting a national culture based largely on Malay elements suddenly disenfranchised the non-Malay Malaysians who had culturally coexisted so freely before independence. Although little work has been published on non-Malay performing arts in Malaysia, it is clear that in this arena, too, there has been increased segregation. In her study of the Chinese *Phor Tor* festival in Penang, for example, Tan Sooi Beng suggests that pro-Malay discrimination practiced by the national government has made the local Chinese population more aware of their ethnicity:

> The festival thrives today because it has assumed extra-religious functions so that Chinese of different social and educational backgrounds can relate to it. . . . [It] provides a vehicle for the defence of Chinese rights and the

protection of Chinese culture. For those who feel their identity threatened, the festival becomes an emblem of ethnicity. Thus, the festival draws Chinese of all social ranks together as a "community" where differences are set aside temporarily. (Tan Sooi Beng 1988, 2–3)

While *Phor Tor* has taken on extrareligious functions, secular urban theater has taken on new life in association with it. *Ko-tai,* for example, a stage show combining Chinese and Western popular songs, would not under normal circumstances be considered an expression of Chinese ethnicity. It becomes acceptable, however, when performed in conjunction with sanctioned religious festivals such as *Phor Tor.* Unlike modern *bangsawan, ko-tai* has remained sensitive to the changing needs of its audience: comic sketches deal with the ills of city life, conflict between the generations, and problems generated by increased social mobility (Tan Sooi Beng 1984). In this respect, it resembles the East Javanese form of urban theater, *ludruk* (Peacock 1968). In its new context, *ko-tai* has become a forum for social commentary, giving young and old, rich and poor Chinese a sense of community, while quietly subverting government attempts to invent a national culture.

Calling for a more comprehensive sociohistorical approach to ethnomusicology (see Tan Sooi Beng 1992), younger-generation Malaysian scholars have begun to discuss the ways in which the performing arts have changed over time in response to the government's struggle to create a national culture in a plural postcolonial society. This book continues the ongoing dialogue, complementing in particular the work of Tan Sooi Beng and Mohd Anis Md Nor. Also, following in John Pemberton's (1994, 12) footsteps, it presents a study of "colonial origins, postcolonial recollections, and postmodern possibilities." As real and fictive constructions of self and community interact on the Portuguese Settlement stage, history is gradually reframed, recontextualized, and ultimately rewritten. Attempting to recover a history that has almost completely been erased, I discuss two closely interrelated yet not entirely congruent histories in chapter 1: the history of the people of the Portuguese Settlement and the history of the place in which they live. In the case of the former, the romanticized narrative promoted in the tourist literature (which casts the residents as hardy descendants of gallant sixteenth-century *fidalgos* [Portuguese: "nobles"] and their beautiful local brides) is examined against the actual historical record. In the case of the latter, I describe the particular set of social circumstances from mid-twentieth-century colonial Malacca that led to the creation of the Portuguese Settlement and show how residents, local government, and travel writers are all gradually rewriting this history, building on a "direct link" to the sixteenth century to relocate the village somewhere between a slice of living history and a historical reconstruction.

The title of this book, *D'Albuquerque's Children,* thus reflects not only the importance of ideas about descent for the people of the Portuguese Settlement themselves, but also in a very tangible sense illustrates Pemberton's model: colonial origins in the physical form of Afonso de Albuquerque and his *fidalgos;* postcolonial recollections that nostalgically reframe history, privileging the Portuguese connection at the expense of a more realistically hybridized Malaysian past; and postmodern possibilities—the onstage transformation that turns contemporary Malaysians into the sons and daughters of a fictionalized Portuguese swashbuckler. I have intentionally made a clear orthographic distinction between Albuquerque as a historical figure and as a near-mythical patriarch: throughout the book I refer to the former as Afonso de Albuquerque or Albuquerque and to the latter as D'Albuquerque. I have deliberately chosen the old aristocratic contraction for the latter because it links the romanticized narrative with the more prosaic present—the actual name of the Settlement's main street is Jalan D'Albuquerque, D'Albuquerque Road). Thus the "children" of the title are simultaneously Portuguese descendants located in the historical imagination and, in the case of the majority of the dancers at least, real-life children of the village.

Just as the Settlement was born in the colonial imagination, so too was the performing tradition for which it is now famous. Once again, however, the recent colonial origin of the "tradition" has been almost entirely eclipsed. In chapter 2, the genesis and development of the genre now known generically as "Portuguese dance" are documented, showing that, far from stretching back into the mists of time, the genre was inaugurated on May 19, 1952, at a performance given by upper-class Eurasians for a visiting Portuguese minister. What began as a one-time exotic novelty for one group of people (upper-class Eurasians) was gradually transformed into an artistic vehicle that helped create and consolidate the identity of another group (lower-class residents of the Portuguese Settlement). At the same time, there was a fundamental change in the process of transmission: what had begun as a literate genre learned from books and notation became an oral tradition passed down from one set of performers to the next.

The remainder of the book presents an ethnographic study of the Settlement's imported tradition—a tradition that has transcended its heterogeneous origins to become, like the direct blood link, another bridge connecting the present-day community with its romanticized past. In chapter 3, the focus is on the performers: the moment they step onto a stage, the imaginary world of the Settlement-as-historical-monument is evoked and they are transformed into D'Albuquerque's heirs. In the glare of the spotlights, the musicians and dancers who perform tradition for a living become part of a living tradition. And yet, while appearing interchangeable, each group of performers is unique, with its own history, social structure, and underlying philosophy forged by the personality of its leader.

The songs and dances uncritically accepted as both "traditional" and "Portuguese" are examined in chapter 4. Forming anything but a homogeneous corpus, they are an eclectic accretion of material from all over the Portuguese world and beyond. The stage becomes a crucible in which songs and dances from different times and places are selected and juxtaposed, fluidly linking Malacca with the Portuguese diaspora across both time and space. On the one hand, the eclectic nature of the repertoire means that each song and dance possesses its own past, different parts of which may be recognized by individual members of the audience, thus constructing the diaspora anew in each performance. On the other hand, through repetition, the heteroglot potpourri is gradually being domesticated into a uniquely local repertoire (at the expense of older, hybrid—and thus less ethnically distinctive—traditions). Viewed from this perspective, diasporic connections are not important: a homegrown taxonomy has developed that bears little resemblance to original relationships, and the music and dance, once imported, have become so deeply rooted in Settlement life that the younger generation, like the tourists, see the repertoire as an unbroken tradition stretching back to the sixteenth century.

In chapter 5, we turn to the performance itself, for it is in the act of performance that temporal and spatial distances collapse, allowing the Settlement-as-housing-estate and the Settlement-as-historical-monument momentarily to converge and become one. But the collision between real and imaginary worlds hides a paradox: the past so rambunctiously celebrated is a past that never existed. Instead, the sanctioned space of the cultural show becomes a crucible in which disparate elements meet and together creatively forge a new synthesis. Detailed analysis of a single performance shows how the cultural show, while appearing to represent "authentic" tradition, actually functions as an "arena of hybridization" (Aggarwal 1996). Viewed in this light, Settlement residents have in fact constructed a perfect metaphor for their community, transforming costumes, music, and dance into crucial markers that not only illuminate their community's imagined and actual pasts but also highlight the complex anachronisms of its present.

In the final chapter, I use the example of a real-life social drama to explore some of the ways in which the performing tradition, the marker par excellence of the Settlement-as-historical-monument, is no longer separable from the political exigencies of the Settlement-as-housing-estate. As the community faces its greatest challenge—the projected extension of a massive land reclamation scheme that will effectively destroy the livelihood of the remaining full- and part-time fishermen—it has become clear that the needs of the Settlement-as-housing-estate cannot possibly stop powerful external business interests. Younger-generation community leaders, appropriating the language of ethnography and invoking the Settlement-as-historical-monument, have proposed turning the village into a living museum, complete with replicas of original houses, (newly) out-of-work fishermen demonstrating their crafts, *and* regular cultural shows. In effect, they would be creating what Barbara Kirshenblatt-Gimblett (1998, 7) has called "heritage," "a mode of cultural production in the present that has recourse to the past. Heritage thus defined depends on display to give dying economies and dead sites a second life as exhibitions of themselves." In this imagined world, residents would reinvent themselves yet again, combining elements of both real and imagined Settlements to become actors playing the parts of constructed "natives."

July 1990 Today the Portuguese Settlement is one of the official sights of Malacca, a must on every tourist's itinerary. The more adventurous visitors come in twos and threes, maps in hand and cameras at the ready, to witness a preserved species in its natural habitat. Others come by the busload—huge air-conditioned buses rumbling down the narrow main street, causing the wooden houses to shake and mothers to pull their children away from the big wheels—for a fifteen-minute pause in their half-day tour of the city. Their guides or guidebooks tell the same story: the Portuguese came to Malacca in 1511, were captivated by the local women, and produced a race of Portuguese Eurasians. Their descendants, despite having suffered at the hands of subsequent colonial powers and having been reduced to the status of lowly fisherfolk, have retained the religion, language, music, and dances of their ancestors. It's a charming story, enhanced, no doubt, by the setting: the Straits of Malacca in the background; children squealing as they play by the sea wall; old women wearing Malay-looking *sarong kebayas*, passing the time of day at a nearby coffee shop; and men—some bare chested—crouched in groups of four, leaning against their small wooden fishing boats, playing cards in the shade of an enormous *ketapang* (chestnut) tree as they wait for the tide to turn.

• • •

Most tourists take this scene at face value, snap their photographs, and hurry off to the next sight/site marked on their maps. The few who take time to pause, however, quickly discover that there are, in fact, two Portuguese Settlements superimposed in time and space. One is a rather unusual low-income housing estate, dating from the mid-1920s and essentially the product of colonial whimsy. Within its confines, ordinary children are born, grow up, get married, and struggle to make ends meet, hoping to make life a little better for their own offspring. The other, a romanticized historical monument and tourist attraction, exists in guidebooks and in the imagination. In this Settlement, the extraordinary exotic Other is displayed as a curiosity. By presenting this Settlement as an anomaly, a vestige of a bygone era, contemporary image-makers effectively rewrite its history. Over time, this newly constructed "history" feeds back, affecting accounts (ranging from the oral testimonies of residents to supposedly authoritative government publications) of history as it "actually happened."

In order to understand how these contrasting Settlements coexist and interact, we must gently untangle two rather different histories—the history of the people and the history of the place. The two are obviously interrelated, but despite the tour guides' patter and the "feedback effect," they are not entirely congruent. If we compare different oral and written versions of the history of the people, we discover a fluid narrative, a story about origins, rather than an accurate account of chronological events. Whether storyteller or historian, each narrator weaves an individual tale from a limited number of narrative threads: the arrival of Albuquerque in 1511; the new race created by his *fidalgos* and local women or by Portuguese orphan girls sent to the colonies as brides; their children, granted Portuguese citizenship by a distant king; and the subsequent reversals of fortune at the hands of later colonial powers, most notoriously the Dutch. The romantic heart of the story, however, lies in the direct blood link to sixteenth-century Portuguese adventurers gallantly led by Afonso de Albuquerque, Portuguese Viceroy of India from 1509 to 1515.

With the exception of a few landmark dates—1511, 1641 (conquest by the Dutch), and 1824 (the British takeover)—the passage of time is condensed to create a bridge between Albuquerque and the present. The second history, that of the place, builds upon the first, using it to cast a veil over the Settlement's more prosaic recent colonial past. By appropriating historical authority in the symbolic form of a direct blood link, the place is made to appear equally old and "authentic." In effect, the imaginary Settlement-as-historical-monument eclipses the everyday Settlement-as-housing-estate.

Origins: The History of the People

Although it might seem to be the case from the narrative threads outlined above, Malacca's history does not begin with the arrival of the Portuguese.

On the contrary, when Afonso de Albuquerque conquered Parameswara's city, he captured an unprecedented prize. For over a century, Malacca had been both the capital of a hereditary Malay sultanate and the busiest, most cosmopolitan port in Southeast Asia. Its fame as an international emporium was so great that the traveler Tomé Pires wrote in 1512, "Whoever is lord of Malacca has his hand on the throat of Venice" (Cortesão 1944, 287). Its location, half way between India and China at a narrow point in the Straits of Malacca, was crucial: control of the city meant effective control of the entire South China Sea spice trade. A natural rendezvous for traders from east and west dependent on seasonal monsoon winds, Malacca was crowded with goods, agents, and traders from all over the world. As Pires noted, "in the port of Malacca very often eighty-four languages have been found spoken, every one distinct, as the inhabitants of Malacca affirm" (ibid., 269).

With Malacca secured, Albuquerque immediately set about establishing a permanent presence. He built a walled city protected by a huge fortress called *A Famosa* and attempted to populate it with a resident community loyal to Portugal. To this end, he continued the policies initiated after his conquest of Goa the previous year. First, firmly believing that married men made better long-term citizens than bachelors, he offered incentives to encourage men to settle down in the new colony. As he described the process in a letter from Goa to King Emmanuel:

> We took here some good-looking Muslim women, of white color. Several of our men, well born and gentlemanlike, asked them in marriage, in order to settle in this land. For that purpose, they asked for money, and I had them married, according to the orders received from your Highness, and to each of them I have given a horse, house, land and cattle. . . . All together there will be about 450 souls. (quoted in Silva Rêgo 1959, 35–36)

Next, batches of Portuguese orphan girls, known as *orfãs del Rei* (Portuguese: "orphans of the king"), were sent from Lisbon to marry either Portuguese men or high-ranking locals, the latter typically as a means of cementing alliances. Again, there were incentives: the young women, sent at the expense of the Crown from 1546 on, "were provided with dowries in the form of minor government posts for anybody who would marry them" (Boxer 1961, 58–59). In addition, legislation in the form of periodic royal edicts confirmed that children resulting from such mixed unions had full rights of Portuguese citizenship. Finally, in a short-term attempt to increase the population, Portuguese citizenship was conferred upon all Catholic converts, regardless of race. Although edicts were not always observed in practice, there was general agreement with the royal belief that "religion and not colour should be the criterion for Portuguese citizenship, and that all Asian converts to Christianity should be treated as equals of their Portuguese co-religionists" (Boxer 1963, 69–70).

Quintessential narrative threads of this sort have been woven into the fabric of history; however, all warrant further scrutiny. In purely demographic terms, for example, we have no precise idea of the size or even racial composition of the original community. No statistics exist in regard to the number of Portuguese men who served or resided outside Portugal during the sixteenth and seventeenth centuries. Estimates, such as Boxer's six to seven thousand able-bodied men, generally refer to the entire *Estado da India* (Portuguese: "State of India"), a nexus of Portuguese possessions and trading posts stretching from Sofala on the southeast coast of Africa to Macau (Boxer 1961, 19–20; 1963, 41). On a more local scale, contemporaneous accounts suggest that the number of European-born Portuguese residents in Malacca was relatively small. In 1580, Padre Alexander Valignano, an Italian Jesuit, wrote that the "town was in former times very big and rich, but now is very small, and has 70 to 80 houses of the Portuguese, and two native suburbs, which are mostly Christians, although there are some heathen and Mohammedans" (Texeira 1961, 1:78).[1] By 1613, Godinho de Eredia counted three hundred married men (called *casados*)—excluding the garrison—who lived within the city walls (Maxwell 1911, 12 n. 3). The number had dropped somewhat by the time Captain Barretto de Resende visited Malacca, shortly before it fell to the Dutch in 1641. He mentioned 250 Portuguese married men, but noted that a hundred lived across the river, outside the city walls (ibid., 4; see fig. 1).

It is even harder to estimate the number of Portuguese women. Boxer (1969, 129–31) dismisses the *orfàs del Rei* as demographically insignificant, suggesting that the scheme was at best sporadic, that there were never more than thirty orphans dispatched per year, and that only between five to fifteen were sent as far as Goa. The number who made the arduous voyage from Goa to Malacca was likely even smaller. Of the few hardy women who survived the journey, some died or miscarried in childbirth. Others were "alleged to be virtuous enough, but too old and too ugly to find husbands" (Boxer 1961, 58–59). Still others remained unmarried because potential suitors complained that the official posts were too poorly paid (Boxer 1969, 129–31).

These chance statistics, suggestive as they are, shed little light on the identity of the settlers of Goa, Malacca, and other Portuguese possessions.

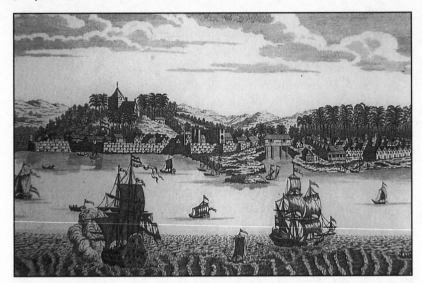

Figure 1 Early etching of Malacca, showing the fortress, St. Paul's Hill, and the "native suburbs" across the river. From Charles Theodore Middleton, *A New and Complete System of Geography* (London, 1777–78).

Romanticized retellings of the story tend to cast the settler-ancestors as heroic *fidalgos* or noblemen. Silva Rêgo (1959, 36) is closer to the mark when he suggests that Albuquerque's "well born and gentleman*like*" husbands were not *fidalgos* but "honest folks, worthy of being forefathers to a new generation." He was probably, however, overgenerous in his assessment of their moral character. Contemporaneous writings clearly indicate that the settlers were mostly soldiers, sailors, and others who had nothing to lose by starting a new life outside Portugal; many of them preferred cohabitation to marriage. In 1580, Padre Valignano regarded the European-born Portuguese residents as unsuitable candidates for admission to the Society of Jesus on the grounds that they were "mostly illiterate pages or soldiers who would have to be taught to read and write" (Boxer 1963, 63). The clearest picture comes from François Pyrard de Laval, himself a Portuguese soldier in India. In 1619, over a century after Albuquerque first sailed into the region, he wrote:

> A vast number of the soldiers are sent to the Indies in exile for their misdeeds: these durst not return before their time has expired. They are sent to Ceilan [*sic*], Mozambique, Malaca and other places to garrison them; these get only their pay without hope of other reward; most of them marry and remain there all their lives. (Pyrard de Laval 1888, vol. 2, pt. 1:124)

Other glimpses suggest that by the mid-seventeenth century, the quality of settlers had further deteriorated to the point that they were "exemplified by 'degenerate' half-castes and frontier whites who were anything but civilized" (Thomas 1994, 2). For example, Fr. Avitabile, an Italian priest resident in Goa from 1640 to 1650, complained bitterly in a letter of December 1645 that "the people who come here from Portugal . . . are the scum of that kingdom, and the most unruly in it, and who cannot stay there. If some of them are *fidalgos,* even they are mostly illegitimate" (quoted in Boxer 1963, 66–67). McGilvray goes further, suggesting that with the exception of Catholic priests, "most of the Portuguese who served in the African and Asian expeditions . . . were exiles and criminals from the great Lisbon prison, the Limoeiro, whose sentences had been commuted to military service in the East" (1982, 238).

In scrutinizing these narrative elements, we should also consider what is *not* told. Apart from the fact that there is no way of knowing whether these former prisoners were in fact hardened criminals or simply poor people who had run afoul of the law, two other crucial potential threads are glossed over in modern retellings. First, the sailors who crewed Portuguese ships and the soldiers in the garrisons—the majority of settlers, according to Pyrard—were not necessarily European-born Portuguese. With a total population of about a million (Boxer 1961, 20), Portugal simply did not have the homegrown manpower to maintain such an extensive seaborne empire. It is more likely that rank-and-file soldiers and sailors were conscripted men or slaves from other Portuguese trading stations in the *Estado da India.* Although there is no consensus among the chroniclers regarding the number of ships or fighting men under Albuquerque's command, we know that he arrived in Malacca with a force comprising roughly 800 Portuguese and anywhere from 200 to 600 "others" described variously as "Malabars," "native foot-soldiers," "native sailors," and even "valiant slaves" (Cortesão 1944, 279, n. 1). Once Malacca was taken, however, it is hard to tell how many (or which) men Albuquerque left to guard and settle the city.

Second, as the royal edicts stipulated, *all* Catholic converts—regardless of race—were considered Portuguese citizens, even to the extent of giving them Portuguese names upon conversion. In the early days, a distinction was certainly made between "white" Portuguese and "native" Catholics; Padre Valignano referred to native Christians in the suburbs, and Godinho de Eredia reported some 7,400 Catholics in Malacca and its environs in addition to the 300 married men *(casados)* already mentioned (Texeira 1961, 1:100). But after Malacca fell to the Dutch, the distinction faded under the twin pressures of periodic religious persecution and continued intermarriage. The terms "Portuguese" and "Catholic" slowly became synonymous, a conflation that has continued to the present. Today there are two Malay names for the Portuguese Settlement: *Kampung Portugis* ("Portuguese Village") and *Kampung Serani* ("Christian Village," from *serani*, "Nazarene," an old synonym for "Christian"). In addition, negative Dutch and British attitudes toward children of mixed-race unions created another disenfranchised demographic group that was quickly absorbed into the local Portuguese community.

Both glossed-over threads have continuing implications for the present-day Portuguese Settlement community. Although residents with Portuguese names predominate, a substantial number of families bear British or Dutch family names. Yet all are Catholic, all speak Kristang, and all describe themselves as Portuguese descendants. Community membership has thus become more a matter of self-ascription than of proven genetic birthright. Portuguese family names are not even a guarantee of legitimate descent, for "names may have come directly from the Church at some genealogical moment or another [and] all we need to know is that *one* ascendant of a given person was an ethnic Chinese or Indian or Malay, and converted to Catholicism upon marrying a Kristang wife, to conclude that the 'direct descent' link to 1511 was broken" (O'Neill 1998, 67). O'Neill's research on kinship patterns in the Portuguese Settlement suggests that the very existence of the community has depended on its ability throughout history to encompass and assimilate outsiders. Even today, maintaining a practice first codified in sixteenth-century royal edicts, the term "mixed marriage" describes spouses of different religious—not ethnic or racial—backgrounds. The defining factor for contemporary community membership is religion, not race.

Transitions

Most retellings of the history of the people condense the passage of time, skipping lightly from sixteenth-century Portuguese Malacca to the present day. Few mention that the Portuguese were the earliest of three colonial intruders. Although the Catholic Portuguese held Malacca from 1511 until 1641, the Protestant Dutch and British controlled it from 1641 to 1824 and from 1824 to 1957, respectively. Those histories that do touch briefly upon Dutch and British times frequently invoke one (or both) of two narrative threads. The first casts faceless Dutchmen as generic conquerors who inflicted a period of religious persecution upon the hardy Portuguese, reduced them to subsistence fisherfolk, forced them into the jungle for secret church services, but were unable to crush their spirit.

The second—more of a witticism than a narrative theme—boasts that the Dutch left their architecture, the British their social order, but only the Portuguese left their living seed (an implied sterility at odds, of course, with the abundance of Dutch and British family names).

With the exception, then, of a few subthemes illustrating Portuguese tenacity in the face of hardship, most versions of the story focus on Malacca's Portuguese heyday, downplaying the city's subsequent three-century decline from major international emporium to quiet backwater. Malacca's demise was presaged by the appearance of occasional Dutch ships at the end of the sixteenth century. The trickle soon became a deluge; lacking the support of a government with colonial inclinations, individual traders combined forces to form the Dutch East India Company (Vereenigde Oostindische Compagnie), a private commercial enterprise chartered in 1602. Giving Malacca a wide berth, the VOC established a rival center of operations in 1619 at Batavia (modern-day Jakarta) on the island of Java. As the Dutch trading empire expanded, the importance of Batavia as its economic and administrative hub also increased. Malacca's importance declined proportionately: its port became obsolete, no longer a staging post on the lucrative trade route; its garrison became a threat, an irritating barrier to Dutch regional supremacy. To secure their position, the Dutch attacked the city with the help of one of the local Malay rulers, the Sultan of Johor. After a protracted siege begun in August 1640, the city finally fell to the Dutch in January 1641. Under Dutch rule, Malacca was little more than a guardpost, protecting ships as they passed through the Straits en route to the new Malay and Dutch entrepôts at Johor and Batavia, respectively (Andaya and Andaya 1982, 68–70). Although oral histories in particular portray the entire Dutch period as a time of intense religious intolerance, official persecution of local Catholics mostly occurred between 1666, when Governor Bort ordered Portuguese Catholics to give up their faith, and 1702, when religious freedom was proclaimed (Hoyt 1993, 48).

A third European colonial power entered the arena in August 1786 when Francis Light took formal possession of Penang on behalf of the British East India Company and King George III. With British commercial interests focused on Penang, Malacca's social and economic decline continued, turning the city into something of a frontier town. A rare eyewitness account from this period is provided by Major Samuel Shaw, the first American consul to Canton, who broke his journey in Malacca from August 17 to 19, 1788:

> Malacca, from being not long since the emporium of the straits and the neighboring coasts, is now dwindled to a mere place of refreshment. It has

been for several years gradually declining, under the ill fortune which has attended the [Dutch] company's affairs throughout India generally; and the recent establishment of the English at Pulo Pinang has given the finishing stroke to its commercial existence.

The women at Malacca are chiefly country-born [Portuguese], and in their dress resemble those of Batavia; though the same cannot be said respecting their manners. They are exceedingly vulgar, and fond of frolicking to an extreme. At their dancing parties they drink vast quantities of beer, wine, and gin, chew betel and areca the greater part of the time, eat a hot supper, then go to dancing again, and seldom leave the house till three or four o'clock in the morning. This mode of conduct renders them libertine to such a degree as to banish from the minds of their male companions every idea of respect or delicacy, I had almost said decency, towards them. (Quincy 1968, 290)

During the Napoleonic Wars (1795–1815), the British consolidated their position by assuming temporary control of several VOC possessions in a bid to prevent them falling into French hands. Their hold on the region was further strengthened in 1819 when Sir Thomas Stamford Raffles, who had strongly opposed the return of VOC possessions on the grounds that the British needed another regional staging post, signed a treaty with a local ruler to establish just such a post on the island of Singapore (Andaya and Andaya 1982, 107–11). Finally, in the Anglo-Dutch treaty of 1824, the two colonial powers agreed pragmatically to consolidate their respective possessions. To this end, a line was drawn through the Straits of Malacca, splitting the Malay world in two. All islands south of the line, including Sumatra and Java, would remain Dutch; everything to its north, including the Malay peninsula and Singapore, would be British territory. Singapore, Malacca, Penang, and Province Wellesley thus became a single administrative unit, the Straits Settlements, governed from India until control was transferred to the British Colonial Office in 1867 (ibid., 122).

We have a clear idea of the size and state of the Portuguese community shortly after the British takeover, thanks to a census submitted to Samuel Garling, the Resident Councillor, by his acting Second Assistant, W. T. Lewis, on June 30, 1827. After mentioning 233 European inhabitants, he turned to the "the Siranies or native Portuguese":

These are the remains of the once large population of Malacca who are now dwindled to no more than 2,289 souls. Although the ancestors of this race originally intermarried with the native women their descendants are now altogether separate and form by Customs and habits a distinct Class. They retain in their countenance, the prominent features of their ancestors although in color, as dark as the natives and are, therefore, very easily distinguished.

These people are all poor and many live in wretched houses erected in that part of Malacca called Banda Hillir. It is by these men that the Inhabitants are so largely supplied with fish—with but few exceptions they have no other employment and are constantly out in small sampans following this precarious livelihood. . . . At Boongha Raya near the river's side they have a decent well built church [St. Peter's Church at Bunga Raya], are biggotted Roman Catholics, and are regularly supplied with Priests who are sent for the purpose by the two colleges at Goa and Macao. . . . They speak a language peculiar to themselves, which may be dominated as Creole Portugueze as the original has been greatly corrupted. (Quoted in Dickinson 1941, 260–61)

With established trading bases in Penang and Singapore, the new British rulers had no interest in reviving Malacca. Its decline complete, Malacca exuded a spirit of genteel decay wonderfully captured by the Victorian lady traveler Isabella Bird, who arrived in Malacca on January 20, 1879. From the deck of a small Chinese passenger boat called *The Rainbow* (captained, incidentally, by a Portuguese Eurasian), she encapsulated the scene in a single sentence: "Very still, hot, tropical, sleepy, and dreamy, Malacca looks, a town 'out of the running,' utterly antiquated, mainly un-English, a veritable Sleepy Hollow" (Bird 1990, 125). The soubriquet appears to have been well deserved: Malacca continued to be known as the "Sleepy Hollow" until the tourist boom shattered its tranquil façade.

Home: The History of the Place

At first sight writing the second history—that of the place—might seem an easier task, for the Portuguese Settlement was only founded in 1926. But residents, local government, and travel writers, each with their own political or economic agenda, are rapidly rewriting this history, building on the "direct link" to the sixteenth century to relocate the Settlement somewhere between a slice of living history and a historical reconstruction. In the Settlement-as-historical-monument, plucky descendants of D'Albuquerque have (against the odds) maintained the customs of their ancestors for centuries. The Settlement-as-housing-estate is barely acknowledged. The façade is so effective that few visitors realize that the Settlement was originally conceived as a haven where the "poor Portuguese" would be resettled and protected from total assimilation. Its instigators were all outsiders—foreign priests, colonial British administrators, and upper-class Eurasians affected by "the appeal of a romantic narrative that nostalgically regrets the destruction of idealized precolonial communities" (Thomas 1994, 15). While many of the upper class shared the same names as the lower-class soon-to-be-Settlers, their daily lives were worlds apart. Despite this, they were ultimately to have a lasting impact on the creation and subsequent development of both the Portuguese Settlement and the performing tradition that developed within it. Consequently, before we can begin to revisit the history of the Settlement, we need to explore the class-conscious social milieu in which it was born. This particular slice of colonial history, pieced together from contemporary newspaper commentary supplemented with histories of the Settlement as written and retold by its residents, is slowly being erased in the postcolonial world and redrawn in the pages of tourists' guidebooks.[2]

Life in the Sleepy Hollow

For much of the late nineteenth and early twentieth centuries, Malacca's Eurasians were divided into two distinct social classes defined by wealth, occupation, and education. The upper class called themselves "Eurasian." They tended to be predominantly of Dutch and British origin, were literate, spoke English, and were employed by the British. Those who were called "Portuguese" were lower class and largely illiterate, spoke Kristang, and mostly worked as fishermen. This class division was certainly not unique to Malacca; most Eurasian communities of the period were similarly split. For example, McGilvray reports the existence of the same deep social divisions in Sri Lanka:

> It has been common practice in discussing the Burghers to distinguish between those of Dutch descent, the "Dutch Burghers," and those of Portuguese descent, the "Portuguese Burghers," or more derogatorily, the "Portuguese Mechanics." . . . The Portuguese are commonly depicted as the great Burgher residuum: poorer, darker, more numerous, and less European. All the Burghers are urbanites, but while the Dutch descendants are strongly represented in clerical work and the professions, the Portuguese are commonly associated with manual trades like blacksmithing, carpentry, and leather-work. . . . The Dutch Burghers, with their bureaucratic jobs, their generally lighter complexions, and their cultivation of English man-

ners, were making a strong show of being Europeans, but the Portuguese Mechanics were visibly more "mixed" in every respect. (McGilvray 1982, 236, 244–45)

In Malacca, pondering the question "What is a Eurasian," one local journalist explained the division thus: "A.1 or Tranquerah Eurasians [are those] who are now or whose parents and forefathers were Government officers and clerks, and whose modes of living, speech, etc., are those of the West," while Praya People, found only in Malacca, "are mostly fishermen and whose twang and habits of behaviour betray their past. They are peaceful and without ambition (save to get a good catch) and so happy and contented with their lot in life" (*MG,* May 9, 1932). As the designations "Tranquerah Eurasian" and "Praya People" suggest, social divisions were reinforced by geographic segregation. Upperclass Eurasians lived mostly in Tranquerah, a wealthy coastal area north of the town center, or, if they were slightly less well off, to the south in Bandar Hilir; the lower-class Portuguese fisherfolk also lived in Bandar Hilir, crowded together at the edge of the sea in an ethnically mixed *kampung* off Praya Lane, just as they were when Lewis made his survey a century earlier (see map 1).[3] Separated by class and residential neighborhood, the two worlds rarely overlapped. About the only common ground was their shared Catholic faith. But, as our journalist observed, even at church there was segregation: "high class Eurasians have the front seats (because they pay pew rents) others [*sic*] behind" (ibid.). Sister Dot, a local nun who grew up in the Tranquerah area, still remembers the segregation:

> There was a very noticeable class distinction within the community. It was particularly noticeable at church, because all the rich Eurasians paid pew rent for the seats in the middle of St. Peter's. The ordinary people had to get there early to get a seat in the side rows. The ones with their own pews would arrive a few minutes before the service began and make a big entrance. . . . There were two really prominent families, the Diaz's and the Rodrigues's. Both had a lot of daughters, who would always come to church wearing identical clothes. The biggest excitement was to see what color clothes each family would wear. Once, the Diaz girls all came dressed in blue. I happened to be wearing a blue dress that day, so I felt very stylish. Then I waited to see what the Rodrigues girls would wear. They all trouped in wearing pure white dresses. So beautiful-*lah!* With a red rose in the small of their backs. No other girls in the church were wearing full white— they looked so beautiful. (SD, July 5, 1998)

Only on the rarest occasions did members of the upper class (even those who had Portuguese names like Diaz or Rodrigues) publicly lay claim to Portuguese roots. One notable instance occurred on the afternoon of April 16, 1929, when members of the congregation of St. Peter's Church turned out to meet the Governor of Macau, Señor Arthur Tagmanini de Souza Barbosa, and his wife, who broke journey for a day on their way back to Europe. In honor of their distinguished guests, leading socialite Mr. R. S. de Souza read a welcome address on behalf of the congregation. With hindsight, de Souza's speech constitutes an early example of the romanticized "history of the people." Professing in overly formal Kristang that they were "honored to descend from the son of Portugal who, through his brave deeds, was the first discoverer of the Orient," de Souza added that "even though four hundred years have passed since Don Albuquerque arrived in this land, we still speak the language and follow the customs of Portugal" (*MG,* April 22, 1929).[4]

UPPER-CLASS SOCIAL LIFE

Most of the time, however, the members of the upper class (or "Upper Tens," as they were nicknamed),[5] identified closely with the British. In this regard, the Upper Tens had much in common with colonial elites elsewhere in the British Empire. Like the Indian Parsi community, they "shaped their ideals and sensibilities and the ideals and sensibilities of their children upon the canons of English colonial culture: its literature, its sociability, its competitive athletics, its pianos, its lace and fitted suits, but also in its dismissal of their countrymen as effeminate, traditional, and lowly" (Luhrmann 1996, 9). But as mixed-race elites like the Sri Lankan Burghers discovered, their admiration was one-sided. "Although the English language and way of life became the model for aspiring Burgher families in the nineteenth century, this group was never permitted to share the status and identity of the British" (McGilvray 1982, 247). No matter how "civilized" they might be, they always remained half-castes in British eyes.

Since the British community in Malacca was relatively small, the Upper Tens provided an alternate elite, whose every social event was carefully monitored in the local press. Until the outbreak of World War II, Eurasian social life revolved around the church, occasional charitable projects (often directed at the improvement of their "poor Portuguese brethren"), concerts, balls, and clubs such as the Malacca Girls' Sports Club or the Eurasian Volunteers. The Sports Club, formed in February 1932, aimed (in typically British fashion) "to provide organised games—hockey, netball, badminton—and to encourage music, concerts, and generally speaking, anything that would make for the physical, intellectual and moral welfare of the rising generation" (*MG,* November 19, 1934). Founding committee members included Mr. H. M. de Souza and Misses Mona Daley, Dorothy de Souza, and Ida Rodrigues (*MG,* April 23, 1933), young ladies who were the cream of Eurasian society. Ida Rodrigues, in particular, often figured in the local news, giving a piano recital here, organizing a concert there. When she married Clement de Silva in 1936, their wedding received the attention usually reserved for a Hollywood starlet.[6] If the Sports Club provided a healthy social outlet for young ladies, the Eurasian Volunteers fulfilled a similar function for young men. Part of the city's defense, the Malacca Volunteers were divided along ethnic lines into four companies: A-Company (European), B-Company (Chinese), C-Company (Malay), and D-Company (Eurasian). Reconvened in 1923 by A. J. Minjoot and H. M. de Souza, D-Company functioned more as a social club than a paramilitary fighting unit.[7]

Concerts, balls, and vaudeville-type variety shows were an important part of the Upper Tens' social world. Staged regularly by both the Sports Club and the Volunteers, they not only provided popular entertainment for the local Upper Tens community but also linked them to colonial elites throughout the British Empire. The young women of the Sports Club, in particular, had organized and participated in such shows since their days at the Convent School in Tranquerah. For example, one notable two-hour performance—given at the school on June 23, 1928, in honor of Don José da Costa Nunes, Bishop of Macau—included songs, duets, recitations, a violin duet, flag drill, monologue, and a short play. All the items were in English (despite the nationality of the guest of honor), and piano accompaniments, when needed, were provided by Ida Rodrigues. The most unusual item on this particular program was a "coon song" performed by seven older girls "dressed like niggers with their faces blackened, [who] created quite a lot of fun" (*MG,* June 25, 1928). Many of these same girls organized the first Sports Club variety show shortly after the club was formed. On this occasion their program included a Spanish Tambourine Dance, a Tango exhibition, and a Hawaiian hula dance. The Eurasian Volunteers organized similar concerts. One such performance included "the old war favourite 'Pack Up Your Troubles In Your Old Kit Bag'" as rendered by Mr. F. J. Scully, a set of Hawaiian songs performed by "Messrs. Scully and Theseira, to the twang of guitars and mandolins," and—showing the close connection between the two clubs—a special guest appearance by the young women of the Sports Club, who performed their Tango number, judged by the reviewer to have been "one of the most delightful things ever witnessed" (*MG,* April 23, 1933).

In Malacca, as in the rest of the British colonial world, the splendid gaiety continued unabated to the eve of World War II. An Easter Dance held on Sunday April 17, 1938, for example, drew a large number of the most prominent Upper Tens families including Capt. and Mrs. Minjoot, Capt. and Mrs. E. V. Rodrigues, Mr. and Mrs. H. M. de Souza Jr., Mr. and Mrs. C. de Silva, and the Misses Westerhout (*MG,* April 25, 1938). Who attended was as important for the smooth running of Upper Tens society as what was on the program. As outsiders looking in, we clearly see a small number of socially active families with a tremendous influence on the cultural life of the community. Social events of this sort, with their ballroom dance demonstrations and quasi-military vaudeville songs, were typical fare for any British expatriate or colonial elite community at the time. So, too, were the occasional "exotic" novelties—tango routines, Spanish tambourine dances, Cuban rhumbas, Hawaiian songs, and even "coon songs."[8] Significantly, though, in keeping with their overtly British orientation, in Malacca there was never the slightest Portuguese flavor. Indeed, under normal circumstances, "anything Portuguese was an insult and low. It was meant for the coolies, the laborers" (HSM, July 15, 1991). Visiting diplomats aside, everyday reference to Portuguese roots would not only mark the upper class as little different from their "poor brethren" but also associate them not with Britain—whose culture they celebrated—but with what was then regarded as little more than a third-rate European nation.

POLITICAL LIFE

Although the membership of D-Company and the Girls' Sports Club was undoubtedly Eurasian, both were primarily social clubs and had little impact on organizing Malacca's Eurasians as a politically active community. The years 1934–35, however, saw a nationwide awakening of Eurasian sensibility: Eurasian Associations in other parts of the country became increasingly active, and there was even an attempt to start a national union.[9] Many topical issues of the day, such as the perennial problem of Eurasian disunity, were discussed in the *Eurasian Review,* first produced by the Penang Eurasian Association in July 1934. The national debate was heard even in the Sleepy Hollow, spurring a *Malacca Guardian* columnist who went by the pseudonym "Enquirer" to ask, "Why is there no Eurasian Association in Malacca?" Pointing out that other Eurasian communities had representative bodies that had "done much for the upliftment of their respective communities," he berated Malacca's residents for their political apathy:

> This shows that the members of this community probably feel that there is no necessity for an association of their own. It is certainly creditable to belong to many clubs, but if a community has no association of their own no progress will ever be made. The Singapore Eurasian Association is one to be emulated by the local Eurasians. It is high time that the Eurasians woke up and rallied themselves together. It is then and only then that as a community they will be of any importance. (*MG*, October 22, 1934)

Enquirer's comments and the prevailing spirit of the day seem to have stung the Malacca community into action, for barely a week later a committee was elected to draft rules for an association.[10] Secretary E. W. Howell's press statement showed just how closely Enquirer's admonition had been taken to heart: "our community is lagging behind and will continue to lag, and perhaps sink into nothingness unless an association will support it. . . . We have in our community individuals who are prominent in different walks . . . we have in our midst doctors, lawyers, electricians, engineers, and others who have proved their worth" (*MG*, October 29, 1934). In a second press statement, made after the final reading and passing of the rules, Howell declared the formation of a Eurasian Association a dutiful and loyal act: "If we want the Government and others to assist us, it is our duty first of all to show that we are deserving of assistance. Through the medium of volunteering we can show how loyal we are, how energetic we can be, and how prepared we are to serve at a moment's notice" (*MG*, December 24, 1934).

CHARITY WORK

By the time the first annual report was published the Malacca Eurasian Association comprised 193 members and had subcommittees for sporting, musical, and educational activities. The same report also included accounts of the Association's charity work, much of which was directed at their "poor Portuguese brethren." On February 10, 1935, for example, the Governor of Malacca and members of the Association visited the new Portuguese Settlement. The committee reported that "as a result of this visit, better housing facilities and cheaper rents in the Portuguese Settlement were secured for our needy brethren" (*MG*, March 26, 1936). Such improvements were short lived. By the time of their next visit, the committee reported that "most of the families were in dire need, some having to be content with only one meal a day, while some others are reduced to begging almost" (*MG,* June 29, 1936).

Other charitable efforts were more lighthearted. On May 12, 1937, for example, the Association organized a Sports Day in the Portuguese Settlement as part of a "Coronation Programme for the poorer children of their community who do not attend school." In retrospect, the rhetoric used in the newspaper's account of the day plainly emphasized the gulf between upper and lower classes. On the one hand, a patronizing tone was reserved for the fisherfolk: "Papa and Mamma were not to be left out of the day's fun. . . . Mamma in her gay sarong and kebaya ran 15 yards with a thread and poor old papa with shaking hand tried his best to put the thread through the needle" (*MG,* May 17, 1937). In treating Settlement adults to children's games, we see paternalistic guardians taking charge of their simple, poor relations. This attitude, of course, was not unique to Malacca. In honor of the upcoming coronation of King George VI, upper-class elites all over the British Empire—and even at home— were providing similar public entertainments for lower-class "natives." On the other hand, the Eurasian Association benefactors commended themselves as "gallant workers [who] succeeded in giving their less fortunate brethren such a happy and memorable time" (ibid.). These stereotypes, negative typecasting of the fisherfolk as happy-go-lucky children versus positive reinforcement of wise and benevolent Upper Tens guardians, were commonplace in the rhetoric of the day.[11] That Settlement women wore *sarong* and *kebaya*—typical Malay dress—further marked the distance between the locally assimilating fisherfolk and the British-oriented upper class.

Creating the Portuguese Settlement

This, then, was the social and cultural milieu in which the Portuguese Settlement was conceived. Upper-class Eurasians identified with the British and "saw in their gloves and carriages a civilizing mission that would bring . . . the grace and authority of a morally superior power" (Luhrmann 1996, 4). Prominent members of this native elite were committed to public service, believing it their duty to help others less fortunate than themselves. The poor lower-class community accepted what was offered and continued their perpetual struggle for survival. The Portuguese Settlement was by far the most ambitious of the many charitable projects visited upon the Praya People by the Upper Tens. Eventually independence (in 1957) would effect a major reversal of fortunes: as the Upper Tens faded from the social scene, the Settlement grew into a thriving community in its own right. Over time, history of the place—like the history of the people—began to take the form of a narrative in which certain threads were elaborated by individual retellers. As the two histories interacted in multiple retellings, the narratives began to diverge and two Settlements emerged: the Settlement-as-housing-estate and the Settlement-as-historical-monument. Again, to understand this process, we must revisit another slice of colonial history.

The idea of establishing a reservation was first proposed in 1926 by Fr. Jules Pierre François of the French Mission (St. Francis Xavier's Church). Concerned with the worsening plight of some of his parishioners, particularly those who lived in the overcrowded *kampung* at Praya Lane, where land erosion was causing houses to crumble into the sea, Fr. François brought his plan to the attention of the British authorities. Right from the start, there was something quaintly appealing about the idea of rescuing the "poor Portuguese" from certain oblivion. Even Reginald Crighton, the Resident Commissioner of Malacca, was convinced of the scheme's worth and remarked, "no doubt this community is going downhill, something must be done to help them and put them in a place where they can be saved guarded [*sic*] for future generations" (as quoted in B. Sta. Maria 1982, 130). Nothing was done to improve the lot of the equally poor non-Catholic residents of Praya Lane.

The Settlement-as-Housing-Estate

Land was immediately set aside for the project: twenty-five lots in the district of Ujung Pasir, about a mile from the old Praya Lane *kampung*, were either requisitioned or acquired for the sum of $30,000 (*Sunday Star*, October 25, 1987; Pintado 1974, 37). Uncertainty over the manner of acquisition and the legal status of the land has resulted in a continuing dispute between Settlement residents and successive British and Malaysian governments.[12] This dispute has become one of the enduring issues in the history of the Settlement-as-housing-estate. Despite initial enthusiasm on the part of the authorities for realizing their whimsical notion, time passed before any real action was taken. Among other difficulties, the land, which was located in the middle of a large mangrove swamp, had to be cleared and drained. Reclamation, undertaken by the public works department, started in 1930 and was completed by 1933 (Chin 1967–68, 2). Finally, on October 2, 1933 the *Malacca Guardian* informed the general public that the Portuguese Settlement Committee was ready to consider applications from potential residents. The rules and regulations concerning occupancy, drawn up by the committee and approved by the Resident Councillor on May 25, 1933, were also published:

> The object is to provide land (such land having already been marked out into lots) on which the poor descendants of the Portuguese Settlers in Malacca prior to British occupation, and other poor Eurasians as may be approved by the Committee of Management, may erect dwellings.
>
> The affairs of the Settlement shall be managed by a Committee consisting of the Collector of Land Revenues (Chairman), the Parish Priest of St. Francis Xavier, the Parish Priest of St. Peter, the Senior Engineer, Mr. D. Theseira and Mr. R. S. de Souza.[13] This Committee is appointed by the Resident Councillor, Malacca, to whom there shall be a right of appeal in all matters. . . .
>
> APPLICATIONS: Applications for lots shall be in writing to the Honorary Secretary (who shall be a member of the committee), and he shall keep records of all applications and subsequent action thereon. Approval or otherwise to be at the discretion of the Committee.
>
> CONDITIONS OF OCCUPATION: Occupants will be tenants at will, and no title will be issued. Rents and assessments due to Government and the Municipality shall be paid regularly at the proper time. Rental for lots will be $1.00 a lot per year and shall be due and payable on the 1st day of January each year to the Collector of Land Revenue at the Land Office, Malacca.
>
> BUILDINGS: All buildings proposed for erection must be approved by the Committee and the Municipality. An approved type plan for attap houses [wooden houses with roofs made from dried *attap* palm leaves] will be provided to suit applicants as a guide but approved applicants may submit their own plans for approval. No brick or permanent buildings will be allowed, except with the permission of the committee and the approval of the Resident Councillor. . . .
>
> No transfers of permits or licenses to occupy lots will be allowed, but a tenant may transfer his rights to any other occupant approved by the Committee, and the Secretary shall make the necessary record in his Register, and a fresh license to occupy will be issued to the new occupant. (*MG,* October 2, 1933)

Today few people question the positive effect of moving the fisherfolk from their ethnically mixed environment into a singular enclave. There must have been some skeptics at the time, though, for the local paper published a defense of the project that was not only spirited but that also began to romanticize the inhabitants: "Whatever the critics may say, the scheme is a commendable proposition, and those who were instrumental in bringing it about deserve the thanks of the Portuguese community. The descendants of such a virile race ought certainly to be preserved from the onslaught of time. A Settlement of this kind is the only practical way of doing it" (*MG,* October 30, 1933). But doubters remained. Even forty years later, Fr. Manuel Pintado, a Portuguese priest resident in Malacca from 1948–93, wondered "whether it was good for those people to be together and settled there. One thing is certain, the formation of the Portuguese Settlement gave the people a strong feeling of belonging. . . . But still, the doubt remains, whether it would not have been better to have left them living side by side with the rest of society" (Pintado 1974, 38).

Criticisms aside, the Settlement was ready for its first residents by 1934. Road names were suggested and approved at a meeting of the planning committee meeting on August 17 (B. Sta. Maria 1982, 156–57). Most commemorated locally significant Portuguese historical figures: Afonso de Albuquerque, Godinho de Eredia, Diego Sequeira, Ruy de Araujo (originally and ever since misspelled as D'Aranjo), and Hieronymous Teixeira.[14] At some point during the preliminary planning, a village headman or *Regedor* (from the Portuguese *reger,* "to govern, rule") was appointed to represent Settlement residents and liaise with the committee.[15] Finally, the first residents moved into the Settlement in 1935. Despite the large number of initial applicants and friendly encouragement from Fr. Coroado, other residents were slow to move in. The prime reason for the poor response was that houses had to be erected at the owner's expense and—being mostly subsistence fishermen—few could afford construction costs. Undeterred, the British authorities intervened again and built ten houses along Texeira Road, which they rented out at nominal sums. This pilot scheme proved so successful that a further fifty-four government houses were erected over the next few years (de Silva n.d., 5).

SETTLEMENT SOCIAL LIFE

In contrast to the well-documented glamorous social activities of the Upper Tens, the drudgery of the fisherfolks' daily lives was of little interest to the local press. Occasional mention of the Settlement was made in the local paper, but it was usually in conjunction with Upper Tens' charitable projects. In 1937, for example, the *Malacca Guardian* proudly announced that "Since the removal of the poor fisher folks from Praya Lane to the Portuguese Settlement in April last year only one death occurred" (*MG,*

April 5, 1937), as if the new environment was responsible for increased longevity. Settlement weddings, dances, and festivities, however, rarely received a mention. Although little is known of musical activities from contemporaneous accounts, older residents remember that *branyo* dances and *mata kantiga* song duels were standard fare at social events.[16] These traditional but distinctly hybridized genres, the women's preference for *sarongs* and *kebayas*, and the concern of Settlement founders to protect the people from complete assimilation, all suggest that—language and religion apart—the daily life of Settlement residents was more Malay than Portuguese.

Occasionally miniature portraits of Settlement life surfaced, almost buried amid more mundane demographic information. For example, we know from a speech made by Claude da Silva to the Legislative Council of Singapore on February 12, 1940, that "the Government has 62 houses let at $2 per month and there are 14 private-owned houses in the Settlement. There are 92 male adults and 80 females, 120 children under 10 years of age and 44 between ages 11 and 15. Of the male adults 49 are fishermen and 15 fishmongers" (*MG*, February 19, 1940). By 1952, the population had increased substantially, although the number of houses had not: there were "78 wooden houses covered with dried palm leaves—*attap*—housing 557 Portuguese descendants, the majority of whom are fishermen or petty clerks" (Agência Geral do Ultramar 1954, 15).[17]

GETTING ORGANIZED

The postwar era was a period of simultaneous expansion and contraction: expansion, because the rank-and-file Volunteers returned from active duty, the building program continued (though at a slower rate), new residents moved in as soon as houses became available, and families grew rapidly; contraction, because the government repossessed the first of several portions of land, thus reducing the total size of the Settlement. As the number of houses and residents increased, a sense of solidarity began to develop and physical improvements were made to the Settlement (see fig. 2). *Attap* roofs were replaced with corrugated zinc between 1952 and 1956. Sand and mud floors were concreted over in 1955 (with cement donated by the Rural and Industrial Development Authority, RIDA). Electricity was supplied by 1957 and running water, piped to individual homes (fig. 3), was widely available by the late 1960s.[18] Finally, for the sum of M$280 (donated by RIDA and the Social Welfare Lotteries Board), a community hall was built by a Settlement carpenter and his family in 1961 (Chin 1967–68, 9, 43).

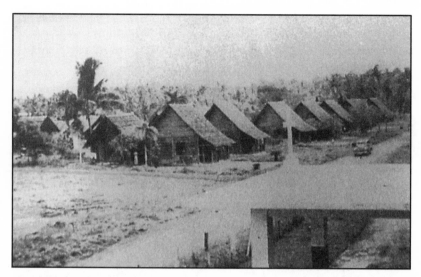

Figure 2 View of the Settlement in the early/mid-1950s. This picture was taken from the balcony of Sacred Heart Convent School before the *attap* roofs were replaced with corrugated zinc. Collection of Sebastian de Silva

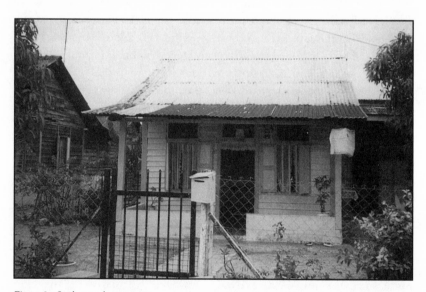

Figure 3 Settlement house, 1991.

As community spirit grew, self-help organizations were established to look after the welfare of residents. One of the earliest such organizations dealt with the issue of funerals. As then Settlement Secretary George Bosco Lazaroo tells the story, it was common practice for a relative (usually a son) to solicit contributions from neighbors and perhaps even from the deceased's workplace to help meet funeral expenses. After one case of a resident passing around the hat at his government office, Lazaroo overheard some colleagues make disparaging comments about the way the Portuguese had to beg to bury their dead. Fueled by his embarrassment, Lazaroo decided to find a better solution (GBL, June 9, 1991). The result was a Funeral Association founded in February 1952 by Lazaroo and *Regedor* Paul de Silva. Aiming "to benefit the poor residents of the Portuguese Settlement in particular," the association had an entrance fee of M$1.00 and a monthly subscription of 50 cents, which entitled all members of the subscriber's family to a funeral benefit of M$40 (A La Bosco 1968, 440).[19]

Even the youngsters began to organize themselves. In 1959, *Regedor* de Silva's son Patrick and Peter Menab (a Malay convert who briefly lived in the Settlement) founded the Portuguese Settlement Youth Club (PSYC). Menab left the Settlement before the club was officially registered, and Cyril Sequerah took over as its first president (de Silva 1990, [6]). In the mid-1960s, during the presidency of Freddie Scully, a rock band and later a dance group were added to the more typical youth club activities—sports events, socials, film shows. Many senior present-generation musicians cut their professional teeth as members of the PSYC rock band, The Zealanders.[20] The organizers of the PSYC were the first generation to grow up in the Settlement; the club continued until they outgrew it.[21] As they married and had their own children, their sense of priorities changed. Some moved away from Malacca, others emigrated, but of those who stayed, many continued to remain active in community affairs.

THE LAND DISPUTE

One central issue has dominated the history of the Settlement-as-housing-estate since the mid-1950s. Always described singularly as "the land dispute" or "the land dilemma," it is actually a complicated series of confrontations between residents of the Portuguese Settlement and two governments (first the British colonial administration, later the Malaysian government) over the status and integrity of their land. In the early years, the ongoing dispute proved an important means of generating solidarity and reinforcing community identity in the face of external threats to the Settlement. By the late 1980s, however, it turned into a divisive issue as battle lines were drawn within the community. The ensuing factionalism—a negative development with continuing repercussions—was nevertheless indicative of the growth of the Settlement as a political community.

The seeds of the dispute were sown unwittingly by the British in April 1949, when, with all good intentions, the Resident Commissioner's Office decided to improve educational opportunities for Settlement children. To this end, a plot of Settlement land measuring about two acres was allocated to the Canossian Sisters for the purpose of building a convent school.[22] Since foreign-based institutions could not own freehold property in colonial Malaya, the Canossian Order was given a 99-year lease for its subdivision (Lot 287) of the original lot (Lot 248). Before long, the Chief Surveyor of Malacca noticed the discrepancy: according to his register, Lot 248 was freehold but its only subdivision was not. He asked the Collector of Land Revenue, Mr. P. R. Lewis, to remedy the anomaly by declaring the entire property crown land, which the latter did in a memo dated August 20, 1949.[23]

Briefly, this capricious change had two major consequences. First, the loss of freehold status meant that the government could repossess portions of the Settlement at will for other purposes. This happened on three further occasions over the next fifteen years: in 1953, for Customs Department staff quarters; in 1962, for a proposed Lasallian Brothers trade school; and in 1964, for Fisheries Department staff quarters (see map 2, below on p. 74).[24] Second, because they no longer lived on freehold land, residents were issued Temporary Occupation Licenses (TOL) for the nominal sum of M$1.00. A continuing irritant ever since, the TOL problem flared up on two further occasions. In 1976 the government offered to replace TOLs with ninety-nine-year leases for sums ranging from M$300 to M$400. Fifty-six households opted to accept the leases; the remainder continued to pay TOL rents. Over a decade later, on July 27, 1987, the problem surfaced again when the government offered leases to those residents still holding TOLs. This time, however, sixty-year leases were offered at considerably higher prices, ranging from M$1,100 to M$2,000. Twenty-one households complied, leaving 41 remaining on temporary licenses either because they could not afford the new assessments or because they refused on principle to buy leases for land they felt was rightfully theirs (*The Star*, August 20, 1987; *Sunday Star*, October 25, 1987).

The first lease controversy became the touchstone for active community political protest. On October 29, 1977, a five-member residents' committee presented Malacca's Chief Minister, Datuk Setia Hj. Ghani with a memorandum on the subject. With a general election looming in mid-1978, local government officials began to discuss the possibility of making the Settlement a Portuguese reserve and even allowed Bernard Sta. Maria, then an opposition member of the State Assembly, to put forward a draft Private Members Bill to this end (J. Sta. Maria 1994, 30–32, 35).[25] Once the election was won, the new Chief Minister predictably "requested the withdrawal of the Private Members Bill . . . as a gesture of goodwill," promising positive action at a later date (B. Sta. Maria 1982, 142).

Although political avenues led nowhere in this instance, the experience of organized political protest was valuable in dealing with the next land dispute-related challenge. In late July 1979, news was leaked that the Customs Department planned to demolish its existing staff quarters and replace them with a high-rise apartment building. This time, organization was swift. On August 2, the *Regedor* held a general meeting and called for volunteers for an action committee to mobilize the wider Eurasian community and to create national awareness of the problem. This time they changed both tactics and rhetoric. Their argument was simple: the Portuguese Settlement was the only place in which a unique culture survived. If residents were outnumbered by non-Portuguese Eurasians, its integrity would be compromised and the community would be destroyed. In a speech made at that meeting, Bernard Sta. Maria showed just how important the Settlement had become as the focal point for the survival of the entire Portuguese Eurasian community. His speech is equally important in retrospect, because it marks the beginning of the elision between the history of the people and the history of the Settlement:

> The Portuguese Settlement is the last bastion where our cultural heritage can continue to be preserved and perpetuated. . . . If the Portuguese Settlement is erased from the map we would become mere nomads, floating from place to place and soon like the gypsies of old, we would disintegrate, with only a name-tag to identify us from whence we originated. As a community of Portuguese descendants, we would cease to exist because a community can only claim to be a community if it possesses a culture, a heritage and an identity. For this to exist we must live in a homogenous environment and the Portuguese Settlement is the only area where such

an environment exists. You cannot perpetuate a community if they have nowhere to organise their festivals, their language is not used in dialogue and their numbers dwindle with the passage of time. (B. Sta. Maria 1982, 147–48)

Four days later, a "Save the Portuguese Community Committee" (SPCC) was formed. Significantly, it was the first time that the word "community" was used in the title of any official Settlement body. The committee's aims were twofold: "to awaken the consciousness of the Malaysian Portuguese descendants on the need to consolidate and to contribute whatever they possibly can to preserve the community's Culture, Identity and Heritage [and] to do research and collect up to date data on the Historical background of the Community" (SPCC, Research Division 1979, 40–41). Barely two weeks later, on August 19, the new committee presented a seminar on the history and evolution of their community. Historical research became a weapon: indigenous retellings of the narrative in the form of formal papers presented by Bernard Sta. Maria, Patrick de Silva, and Rachel Sta. Maria stressed the authenticity of the community, and by extension, the authenticity of the Settlement (see B. Sta. Maria 1979; de Silva 1979; and R. Sta. Maria 1979). Organized protest, appeals to government officers and to Eurasian associations throughout Malaysia, and media attention all had the desired effect—the Customs Department abandoned its planned apartment block.

The united front crumbled when the lease issue resurfaced in late July 1987 followed almost immediately by Bernard Sta. Maria's sudden death. At first the protest seemed to be going well: by the end of August a Land Action Committee led by Bernard's youngest brother, Joseph, was formed. Appeals for support were sent to Eurasian associations around the country (J. Sta. Maria 1987) and even the Chief Minister stepped in to reassure residents that "the Settlement would be protected even if they do not obtain freehold status on the land they are now occupying" (*NST,* October 27, 1987). But in the midst of this struggle, a split occurred between the Land Action Committee, supported by a large number of residents, and a small faction led by *Regedor* Michael Young and former Secretary George Bosco Lazaroo. The former faction opposed the government line and demanded nothing less than confirmation of freehold status; the latter preferred a less confrontational approach, working through government channels to have the land declared a historical zone. Unhappy over the *Regedor's* handling of the situation (perceived by some as a sellout), residents presented him with a petition of no confidence and formed a committee to look into the possibility of electing a new *Regedor*. The argument raged in the Settlement and the local press for about a month. In the end, Young's resignation was overruled by the state government, which insisted that he form a subcommittee to assist him in carrying out his duties. A new non-representative *Regedor*'s Panel replaced the elected Residents' Association as the primary guardian of the day-to-day running of the Settlement, and the freehold/lease issue was never resolved.

The Settlement-as-Historical-Monument

Three years later, completely out of the blue, the Settlement was placed under the jurisdiction of the Malacca Preservation and Conservation of Historical and Cultural Heritage Enactment of 1988. In effect, it became an official historical monument, and Chief Minister Tan Sri Abdul Rahim Tamby Chik assured residents that they "need not fear anymore as the settlement will remain there forever now that it is protected by the enactment" (*NST,* August 23, 1990). This unexpected designation owed more to a new factor—the growth of the tourist industry in Malacca—than to any real attempt to resolve the land dispute. The government's action was motivated primarily by the significance of the Portuguese community as an asset, a crucial part of the historical image it had so successfully packaged. By certifying the Settlement as a monument and placing it (and its inhabitants) alongside genuine relics such as the ruined church atop St. Paul's Hill, the Santiago Gate (fig. 4), and the old Dutch Stadthuys, the government has authenticated the imaginary Settlement, conferring upon it an aura of timelessness.

This security, however, was short lived. Since the mid-1990s residents have been faced with a new chapter in the land dispute and a perhaps insurmountable challenge: development. State government plans to reclaim the last remaining vestige of Malacca's natural seafront will effectively landlock the Settlement and destroy the livelihood of the remaining full- and part-time fishermen. The state government is in a quandary: on the one hand, tourism is its most profitable industry and the Settlement has become a central feature of the package; on the other, dreams of progress, development, and huge gleaming seafront condominiums are seductive. The scale of the project is enormous:

> A M$130 million ($53 million) land-reclamation project threatens to cut off this tiny Portuguese enclave from the sea, a move many residents feel would imperil its very existence.... Olympia Land, a Kuala Lumpur Stock-Exchange-listed company has won the contract to reclaim the land at the

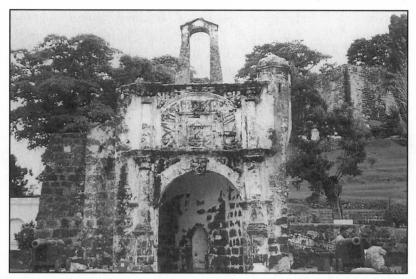

Figure 4 Santiago Gate. The only surviving part of Albuquerque's fortress, *A Famosa.* The ruined church on top of St. Paul's Hill can be seen in the background.

community's seafront. Olympia will extend the shoreline by more than 500 metres, pumping silt from the bed of the Straits of Malacca. The new land will be the site of condominiums and a commercial centre. . . .

If the project cannot be stopped, the [Settlement] panel has asked for a 100-metre corridor of land from the existing village to the new seafront. The reply from Chief Minister Datuk Mohamad Zin Abdul Ghani? The settlement can buy the land at market rates of M$30 per square foot, he says. At that rate, the panel calculates, the corridor would cost M$1.3 million ($530,000). But the community can't afford to pay. (Hiebert 1995, 50)

It seems likely that this time the residents of the Portuguese Settlement may be faced with a battle they cannot win. Ecological protests against the destruction of inshore fishing grounds, and hence of the traditional occupation of a small number of fishermen, are worthless in the face of development and massive economic gain. In now traditional fashion, residents have organized a new committee, the Reclamation Action Committee (RAC), to lead the protests. This time, however, articulate and vocal younger residents, spearheaded by Michael Singho and Gerard Fernandis, have advocated a major change in strategy. They feel that the best chance of beating the property-developing tycoons lies not in trying to save the fishermen's dying livelihood but in convincing the government that destruction of the Settlement's seafront would destroy a vital part of Malacca's tourist image. Adopting the language of the image makers, Singho has invoked themes of cultural loss and touristic rescue. By reappropriating the romanticized tourist myth and transforming it into a survival narrative, Singho and his friends once more demonstrate pragmatic Settlement flexibility in the face of adversity. According to Singho,

> the Portuguese heritage plays a significant role in selling Malaysia to tourists abroad. Yet the returns from the industry do not tally with the role their heritage has in it. . . . The full potential of its tourists' wealth, cannot be realized, if reclamation robs it of its seafront influence. Whatever attraction the settlement possessed would start to disintegrate and eventually be replaced with a forlorn look of an abandoned relic. It is rather strange to stifle an established tourist destination of great promise, while seriously engaged in the development of the industry in the state. (Singho in *The Star,* March 3, 1994)

In another context, Singho has also stated:

> Tourists would then miss the treat of watching the wedding scenes, cultural dances and musical performances, with the sea in the background, providing a resort-like scenery. To lose an essential feature of a popular tourist destination is like clearing a National Park of its trees and landscapes. (Singho 1998, 25)

Singho and his peers have joined the elders in their fight because they feel strongly that the loss of the Settlement will result in the dispersal of the community and in the eventual loss of what they see as its unique culture. In addition to the usual consciousness-raising activities, the RAC followed the example of the SPCC, the only action committee to have scored a notable success, and organized another seminar. This time, however, instead of asking residents to prepare historical papers, they went one step further and organized an "International Save the Portuguese Settlement and Heritage Conference," inviting foreign scholars who had done research in the Settlement to present papers that testified to the historical significance of Portuguese Eurasian culture in Malacca.[26] It was a clever tactic: not only was history used to authenticate the people, their language, and traditions, but foreign academics with Ph.D.s were also used to authenticate history itself.

It is questionable whether the reclamation project can be stopped permanently, although the downturn in the Malaysian economy of the late 1990s and an "island concept" fad have provided temporary respite.

However, an interesting possible compromise has been suggested by Michael Singho. Adding an eccentrically postmodern twist to the story, Singho has proposed turning the Settlement into a heritage park, a living museum with replicas of original houses, fishermen demonstrating their crafts daily, and regular cultural shows. By recycling dying industries and past colonial relations in the name of tourism, Singho proposes giving them, in the words of Bruner and Kirshenblatt-Gimblett (1994, 435) "a second life by bringing them back as representations of themselves and circulating them within an economy of performance." Live displays of this sort, whether recreations of daily activities, such as fishermen mending their nets, or staged as formal cultural shows, "also create the illusion that the activities you watch are being done rather than represented, a practice that creates the effect of authenticity or realness" (Kirshenblatt-Gimblett 1998, 55). If Singho's plan were to materialize, not only would Settlement residents become professional actors playing the part of themselves (becoming, in the process, "professional natives"—or in Kirshenblatt-Gimblett's terms—"signs of themselves"), but the imaginary Settlement-as-historical-monument would become real—or at least an imagined version of an imagined past would become visible—and the actual Settlement-as-housing-estate would be rendered invisible.

Two

INVENTING A
TRADITION

September 1990 It's Saturday night in the Portuguese Settlement and the parking lot is packed tightly with vehicles of all
shapes and sizes. The drivers congregate in casual groups, smoking
as they wait patiently outside the Portuguese Square. Inside the
dilapidated cream-colored stone Square with its red tiled roof, you
almost believe you've stepped into old Portugal. The round tables
are full to capacity: people from all corners of the world sit together
talking, laughing, eating, drinking. A gentle sea breeze ruffles the
leaves of a small *ketapang* tree as the incoming tide laps at a low
stone seawall. Against the wall is an empty white stage, its multicolored winking lights promising action. Four musicians casually
climb its steps and start to tune their instruments. With no percep-
tible signal, they break into a waltz and, as the mouthorgan chugs
busily against a lazy violin countermelody, a portly man wearing
a wide-brimmed hat takes the microphone:

> "Well, ladies and gentlemen, a very good evening to one and all,
> and on behalf of the organizers, the State Economic Development
> Corporation of Malacca, I would like to extend a very warm wel-
> come to each and every one of you to this historical city of Malacca
> and, of course, to the Portuguese Settlement. For tonight you are
> here to be entertained with Malacca's own traditional songs and
> dances. . . ."

Freddie Scully is momentarily interrupted as four smiling young
couples ascend the stage and take their places for the first dance.

> "Now ladies and gentlemen, we present you with a very old num-
> ber, an old favorite of ours, a dance I should say more than one
> or two centuries old, and it's still popular in Portugal. Ladies and
> gentlemen, 'O Vira Viroos.' . . ."

As he begins to sing, all eyes are drawn center stage. The dancers of D'Tiru-Tiru Portuguese Cultural Group—the black, white, and red of their costumes becoming blurred against the dark sea—swirl effortlessly to the lilting music.

• • •

This is the image most tourists capture with their flashing cameras and state-of-the-art camcorders and carry back to their distant living rooms. This is how the tiny Portuguese community is known throughout Malaysia and beyond. In the hands of a skilled emcee, music, dance, and costume are as effective as the direct blood link in creating a bridge between past and present. Together they connect the present-day housing estate to the legendary world of D'Albuquerque. Together they generate an aura of authenticity that facilitates the Settlement's transformation into a slice of living history.

Like the Settlement-as-historical-monument, however, this image is another construction artfully crafted from a limited number of narrative threads: the hardy survivors who have maintained the traditions of their homeland in the face of adversity; the music-loving, guitar-strumming Portuguese; the village where everyone loves to drink and dance. Once again, the recent colonial origin of the "tradition" is almost completely eclipsed. To understand the process of invention and erasure fully, we must not only revisit the historical record, accessible primarily through oral testimonies and newspaper reports, but also examine what Keeler (1996, 226) has called the "genealogy of the idea of tradition"—the particular circumstances and needs that converged to precipitate its invention. Such an examination reveals that far from being an immutable tradition passed down through the generations, it is a tradition pragmatically manipulated in response to specific historical moments and changing political exigencies. As we have seen already, Settlement residents have survived—and even prospered—by engaging in an ongoing process of dialectically inventing and reinventing both their community and its history. As we shall see, music, dance, and costumes are the preeminent means by which this has been achieved.

Shadows of Independence: Adapting to a New World

Just as the Portuguese Settlement was born in the imagination of Frs. François and Coroado in 1926, its performing tradition was conceived with the help of another foreign priest, Fr. Manuel Joachim Pintado.

Posted to Malacca in 1948, Fr. Pintado arrived at a time of deepening crisis for upper-class Eurasians. The War was over, the Japanese defeated, and British rule restored, but colonial authority was no longer unquestioned. The British were tarnished heroes after their humiliation at the hands of the Japanese. Throughout the country, thoughts were turning toward independence. Eurasian intellectuals tried to gain a foothold in the emerging order, but their numbers were too insignificant, their demands too great, and their internal conflicts too bitter. As political parties based on ethnic blocs were starting to emerge in 1951, the fledgling Eurasian Union of Malaya collapsed as a political force of any consequence (B. Sta. Maria 1982, 187–93). When the Alliance—the coalition of Malay, Chinese, and Indian parties that dominated politics from pre-independence until 1969—was born in 1952, the Eurasians were left out in the political cold (Nash 1989, 43).

The Malacca Upper Tens were faced with a dilemma: their primary identification centered on the wholesale adoption of British social and cultural values, but with the colonial era drawing to an inevitable close, association with the British was suddenly more of a liability than an asset. A new affiliation was clearly needed, and, in May 1952, a serendipitous visit by Commander Manuel Maria Sarmento Rodrigues, the Portuguese Minister for Overseas Territories, provided just that. Emulating his seafaring ancestors, the minister was in the process of visiting the Portuguese colonies and former territories under his jurisdiction by sailing ship. While there had been other occasional visitors from Macau and even Portugal, Sarmento Rodrigues arrived at the precise moment upper-class Eurasians needed to reinvent themselves. The status of this particular visitor, the scale and timing of his voyage, and the implied linking of Malacca to a wider Portuguese world with a romantic and adventurous past together fired the imagination of upper-class Eurasians. Suddenly the stigma was removed, and it became acceptable—even fashionable—for society Eurasians with Portuguese (and even non-Portuguese) names to identify themselves as "Portuguese."

It was the conjunction of factors that was crucial: a visit thirteen years earlier by the same sailing ship—the Gonçalho Velho—had triggered no similar response. That three-day visit had evoked a typically British response from the Upper Tens, with formal dinners, tennis parties, separate sight-seeing tours for officers and enlisted men, and a church parade by D-Company and the sailors. Despite being "the first time since the Portuguese squadron from Goa sailed away after the surrender of the besieged Portuguese garrison in 1641 [that] a vessel of the Portuguese navy [has] anchored off the Port of Malacca," the occasion produced neither overt declarations of Portuguese identity nor expressions of cultural brotherhood from upper-class Eurasians. The officers and crew of the ship, however, were "specially interested in the inhabitants of the Portuguese Settlement in Bandar Hilir. Many and long were the conversations which took place between the old colonists in the settlement and the sons of modern Portugal" (*MG,* January 9, 1939).

May 1952: The Portuguese Minister's Visit

Thirteen years later, Malacca was a different place. This time the Gonçalho Velho was a catalyst for the legitimation and subsequent expression of upper-class Portuguese identity. The crucial significance of the minister's visit was still remembered by society Eurasians like Horace Sta. Maria, as demonstrated in the following excerpt from a longer interview:[1]

ms: Your family was more on this Upper Tens side?

hsm: Yes, Upper Tens, although we were Portuguese and we moved around with the Portuguese and we spoke the language. But the Upper Tens were those who had such names like Brown or Atkinsons and they don't speak Portuguese. They were the Upper Tens. And somehow or other, Westerhout, of course is Dutch, they were the Upper Tens. Rodrigues, of course with a Portuguese name, but they considered it— what do you call it?—a bit *low* to admit they are Portuguese *until* the visit of the Portuguese minister when they put themselves forward and joined and started the Portuguese dance.

ms: They didn't have any Portuguese dance before that?

hsm: Never anything Portuguese until the minister. Before that anything Portuguese was an insult and low. It was meant for the coolies, the laborers. . . . When this Portuguese minister came to Malacca to visit us, that's when the interest in Portuguese began to come up. It so happened that when the Portuguese minister came to visit Malacca, no one could dance a Portuguese dance. Then Fr. Pintado was here and he wanted to put on something for them. Then he got us Portuguese Eurasians around, with Ida de Silva and her husband, Clement de Silva— they were the pianists—and taught us just one or two dances.

ms: Fr. Pintado taught you how to dance, or somebody else?

hsm: Somebody else, from the book with Fr. Pintado and so on. Just from scratch. They put on the "Tiru Liru" and "O Vira"—two dances only. (hsm, *July 15, 1991*)[2]

If the minister's visit provided stimulation for upper-class Eurasians, May 19, 1952 was a red-letter day for the people of the Portuguese Settlement. Even forty years later, Sarmento Rodrigues's inspection of the Settlement is remembered with pride by older residents. Local papers covered the event, using increasingly stereotypical imagery to romanticize the Settlement and its inhabitants. Dimly remembered past glories were juxtaposed against present modest circumstances in which *sarong* and *kebaya*-clad women and barefoot men broke out into song to express their happiness:

> Today has been a day Eurasians here will never forget. Amid pomp, gaiety and introductions, thoughts flashed back to the 16th century when Portuguese ruled Malacca and when St. Francis Xavier preached here. . . . In the Portuguese Settlement cooking pots remained untouched and fishing boats did not go out today as everyone gave a heart-warming welcome to the Minister and his party. Women of the Settlement turned out in sarong and kebaya, their hair well-oiled with gold plated pins in their buns. Menfolk wore a variety of clothes from palmbeach suits to Hawaiian shirts. Some old men and young boys turned out barefooted, but everyone was there to see and greet with song "Senor Rodrigues," as they called the Minister. (Unidentified newspaper clipping, May 1952)

The minister and his party arrived at the Portuguese Settlement around midday and were received by *Regedor* Paul de Silva and Secretary George Bosco Lazaroo. After the latter gave a welcoming address, a traditional "wedding scene" and a mock *branyo* dance were performed.[3] Later in the afternoon, the minister and his party made their way to the town center for a formal reception given by the upper-class Eurasian community. At first sight, the whole event, organized around afternoon tea, was remarkably British. After tea,

> an exhibition of folkloric songs and dances was presented by the Portuguese community at 4:30 P.M. in the Capitol Dance Hall. It was watched by around 540 Portuguese descendants in addition to civic and military authorities, leaders of Malay, Chinese, and Indian communities, and other prominent Malaccans. Some of the Portuguese descendants had traveled over 70 miles to pay homage to a minister from their old motherland.[4] (Agência Geral do Ultramar 1954, 21)

This time, however, the entertainment was markedly different from anything produced in the old Girls' Sports Club and Eurasian Volunteers days. First, upper-class Eurasians publicly identified themselves as mem-

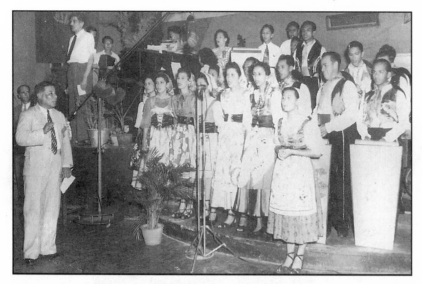

Figure 5 Group photograph from the Capitol Dance Hall tea entertainment, May 19, 1952. Arquivio Histórico Ultramarino do Instituto de Investigação Científica Tropical, Lisboa

bers of a "Portuguese community." And second, the program presented Portuguese songs and dances to a Malacca audience for the first time.[5] Portuguese songs learned from notation, "Regresso ao Lar" and "O Trevo," were mixed with newly composed songs ("Amor mia Amor") and *branyo* tunes ("Ala Banda Esti Banda" and "Jinkly Nona"). (Even though the most popular *branyo* tunes of their "poor brethren" were included, the melodies were neatly harmonized by Horace Sta. Maria and his group, the Tres Amigos.) In addition, two Portuguese dances were performed by a group of Upper Tens, including a number of the leading non-Portuguese Eurasians, such as Ivor Westerhout, Lawrence Minjoot, and Jackie Lewis (see fig. 5):[6]

> "Tiru Liru Liru," was performed by a group of young men and women wearing Portuguese regional costumes. This number raised great interest and deserved much applause for the graceful movements and attractive costumes. . . . The program continued with a popular dance "O Vira," with the dancers appearing again in varied and elegant regional costumes from the Portuguese metropolitan provinces.[7] (Agência Geral do Ultramar 1954, 23, 31)

Although primarily an Upper Tens social event, segregation was not absolute: one item on the program, a Kristang poem, was recited by an eleven-year-old Settlement boy, Master Emmanuel Bosco Lazaroo. In addition,

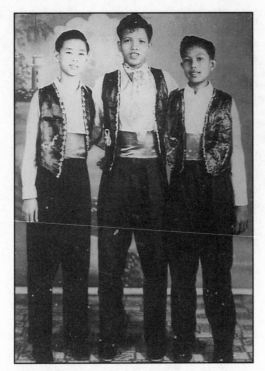

Figure 6   Three Settlement boys (*left to right:* William Tan, Georgie de Costa, Patrick de Silva), ca. May 1952. Collection of Patrick de Silva

according to Patrick de Silva, he and two other Settlement boys sang for the dancers under the direction of Clement de Silva (PDS, October 22, 1990). Considering their age and social status, it is perhaps not surprising that these boys were omitted from the official program and group photograph. A separate picture of the three boys in their Portuguese outfits was taken around this time (see fig. 6).

The Pageant

For some of the older Upper Tens participants, membership in the first dance group was short lived: soon a new project, the Pageant, occupied their attention and organizing skills. Although amateur theatricals of this sort were an established part of the colonial social world, once again it was the scale, timing, and subject matter that made this particular pageant noteworthy. It was part of an ambitious project, a ten-day celebration of the fourth centenary of St. Francis Xavier's landing in Malacca. The celebration drew a large number of visiting dignitaries, including the archbishop of Indonesia, the bishops of Thailand, Macau, and Malacca, the minister for Portugal in Indonesia, and the Swiss consul from Singapore.

A sacred relic was even brought from Macau and carried in a monstrance by Ida's brother, Fr. Lancelot Rodrigues, who returned home as the bishop of Macau's representative (*SS,* March 13, 16, 21, and 23, 1953).

Based on the life of St. Francis Xavier, the Pageant was the center-piece of the celebration. It was an enormous production, involving most of the leading lights in the Eurasian community, requiring the cooperation of all the Catholic churches in Malacca, and using over sixty costumes (valued at M$9,000) loaned to Fr. Pintado by the Portuguese government. According to Theodore Moissinac, who played the part of St. Francis, over two hundred performers were involved, including children from local Catholic schools and Settlement people (the latter, predictably, playing the parts of lower-class soldiers and sailors).[8] Members of the Upper Tens, of course, played leading roles: old photographs show Lawrence Minjoot and his wife as king and queen of Portugal, Jackie Lewis as an officer, and Ivor Westerhout as a *fidalgo.* A minuet and other European stately dances were included in the Portuguese court scene, accompanied by an orchestra of local school children. Portuguese folk dances arranged by Arthur Sta. Maria were also included, although these were only accompanied by his brother Horace on guitar and a chorus of small boys and girls (TM, July 31, 1991). The four ticket-only performances given on the lawn of the British Residency in the shadow of St. Paul's Hill were watched by an estimated 35,000 spectators.

The minister's visit and the Pageant both mark a strategic embracing of Portuguese cultural and historical themes on the part of the Upper Tens. In a pragmatic attempt to disassociate themselves socially and culturally from the British, they found an effective way to melt into the postcolonial environment. It was an ideal compromise: a ready-made "tradition" that was recognizably European but not British. The historical link with Portugal generated prestige, status, and historical legitimacy (not to mention adding a certain swashbuckling romance) without awakening recent colonial memories. At the same time it linked them cosmetically with a disadvantaged local group, the poor Portuguese fisherfolk. First a novelty, later a fashionable activity, and finally an acceptable marker of non-British European identity, Portuguese music, dance, costumes, and historical themes together constituted a symbolic way of negotiating their new position in a changing world.

Transitions: Passing the Torch

While the Pageant consumed the attention of older society Eurasians, a few younger members, led by Arthur Sta. Maria (Horace's brother) and

Christie Rodrigues (Ida's sister), remained enthusiastic about Portuguese folk dance and continued to organize groups to perform for special occasions. At this early stage their repertoire was small. Ruy Cinatti, Fr. Pintado's friend, had taught them only three dances: "O Vira Vamos," "Tiru Liru Liru," and "O Malhao." According to Christie Rodrigues,[9] soon after the minister's visit she found a book on Portuguese folk dance at Lim's Bookstore. The book contained the music and steps for four more dances, which they recreated from the notation, adding their own variations (CRK, March 19, 1991).[10]

During the 1950s there was a gradual expansion of repertoire. New dances were acquired from a variety of sources: some were recreated from written notation, others were set locally. Around this time, Christie Rodrigues made the first of many trips to Portugal. After the Pageant, she and Irene Nunis were selected by Fr. Pintado to represent Malacca at a church-organized jamboree attended by youths from all over the Portuguese world. Christie recalled that during the huge cultural exchange they spent two or three months traveling around Portugal (CRK, March 19, 1991). The experience not only fueled her enthusiasm for Portuguese folk music and dance but also gave her the opportunity to observe diverse regional styles and to learn new dances.[11]

By the mid-1950s, it was increasingly common to find Portuguese Eurasians of different class backgrounds dancing together. The Upper Tens found themselves in a difficult position as independence approached: their British role models were gone and upper-class ways were no longer acceptable. The same was happening to colonial elites all over the Empire. As Alex Van Arkadie remembers of the situation in Sri Lanka, for example,

> the Burgher people had only one or two leaders to represent them in the local political arena. When the issues of a majority language, community, religion began to be debated in parliament the Burghers realized that they were socially being humbled to their knees. I recall the humiliation most of our Burghers suffered. Many left for residential status offered in English-speaking countries of the British Commonwealth, viz., Australia, Canada and the United Kingdom. (Pers. comm., May 25, 1999)

In Malacca, too, those who could not adapt to the new world emigrated to Singapore, Australia, or even England. Those who remained of necessity forged closer links with residents of the Portuguese Settlement. Arthur Sta. Maria, for example, although a member of the Upper Tens, began to train a group of dancers in the Settlement in 1954 or 1955 (pers. comm., June 21, 1999; see figs. 7 and 8).[12]

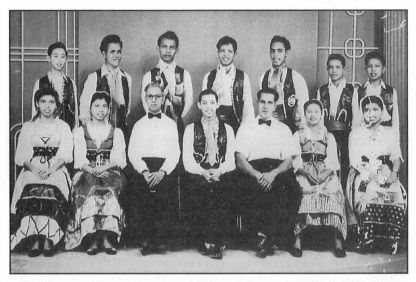

Figure 7 First Settlement dance group, ca. mid-1950s. Collection of Patrick de Silva

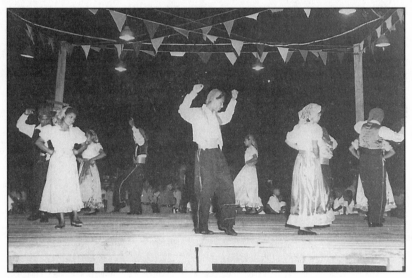

Figure 8 First Settlement dance group in performance, ca. mid-1950s. Collection of Aloysius Sta. Maria

Dancing in the Portuguese Settlement

The dance group continued quietly in the Portuguese Settlement, attracting a steady stream of young members. A typical Christmas program from the mid-1950s shows variety concerts similar to those previously organized by the Upper Tens but with a clear Portuguese flavor. Comic relief was provided by Denny Pestana, the Settlement clown and former *bangsawan* theater performer. One novelty item reminiscent of the Girls' Sports Club shows and still fondly remembered by former dancer Josephine de Costa (née Theseira) was a hula dance performed by Gerard Sta. Maria, wearing only a grass skirt and accompanied by a chorus singing "Rhythm of the Islands" (JTC, July 1, 1991).[13] The *branyo*, the favorite social dance of Settlement residents (described on the program as a local folk dance), was used from these early days to conclude performances, adding a distinctively Settlement touch to the variety format. Audiences for such concerts were, according to George Bosco Lazaroo, mostly outsiders, people from all over Malacca, including colonial officials (GBL, June 1, 1991).

It was not long before the variety concert format was further modified and non-Portuguese items were dropped from the repertoire altogether. The emcee's introduction to a 1956 program described eight Portuguese songs performed by Horace Sta. Maria, the Tres Cavalieros, and the Settlement Youths, interspersed between four dances.[14] George Bosco Lazaroo, emcee on this occasion, was careful to inform his audience that the songs and dances were "imported from Portugal" (Lazaroo 1956). As before, the performance ended with a local *branyo*, but this time Lazaroo announced that "the boys section of the Youth Movement headed by Denny Pestana the Clown will invade the guests territory and demand from you a dance. I hope ladies and gentlemen you will accept their invitation to dance the local branyo" (ibid.). Programs have changed little since 1956: there are more dances and fewer songs these days, but the same basic mix is observed, often concluding with a *branyo* in which the audience may be invited to participate on stage.

The Portuguese Settlement Youth Club

The dance group continued for some years, but performances were infrequent, and, according to Horace Sta. Maria, the group was in virtual hibernation by the mid-1960s (HSM, July 15, 1991). Its decline in activity coincided with the growing vitality of Settlement organizations, including a dance group sponsored by the Portuguese Settlement Youth Club (PSYC). Run by club president Freddie Scully, the main instructors were Joe Lazaroo and Walter Sequerah, both experienced dancers from the early days.[15] Scully, too, had previously danced, but only after 1957 when he returned from working in Singapore. The Youth Club group capitalized on the slowly growing commercial value of Portuguese music and dance in Malacca. While earlier groups had always performed for outsiders and occasionally been paid for their efforts, the PSYC group was formed in response to a specific contract. According to Scully, an American Express agent wanted to hire a group to give lunchtime shows for tourists two or three times a week: when the contract expired, the group was disbanded (FJS, June 26, 1991).

To this point, repertoire and format of performance had remained fairly stable: a few new dances were learned, the *branyo* was added as a concluding item, and audience participation was introduced, but otherwise little had changed from the earliest days of Clement de Silva's group. Still acknowledged as having been imported from Portugal, it was not yet packaged as part of a uniquely Malaccan cultural heritage. This started to change as the Upper Tens faded from the social scene and the formerly lower-class Portuguese descendants—residents of Praya Lane and the Settlement—became more active and concerned with fostering a growing sense of community. This societal shift effected two crucial changes. First, there was a complete transformation of function: what had begun as a one-time exotic novelty, a means of tapping into a glorious past for one group of people (the Upper Tens) was transformed into an artistic vehicle for the creation and consolidation of contemporaneous community identity for another group (residents of the Portuguese Settlement). And second, there was a fundamental change in the process of transmission: what had begun as a literate performing genre learned from books and notation became an oral "tradition," passed down from one set of performers to the next.[16]

Stormy Waters: Adjusting to Political Change

The decade following independence was a period of community building both in the Settlement and across the nation. With a certain measure of community identity established by the late 1960s, Settlement residents began to look outside themselves. In a first attempt to ignite this new-found spark of political awareness, Bernard St. Maria and a group of mostly Praya Lane residents established the Portuguese Cultural Society in 1967. Not a Settlement resident himself, Sta. Maria intended the society to be both a vehicle for uniting all Malacca's Eurasians and an interface between them and the wider Malacca populace.[17]

The Portuguese Cultural Society

Echoing the sentiments of Resident Councillor Reginald Crighton forty years earlier, the Cultural Society was the first home-grown organization to assert self-consciously that Portuguese Eurasians shared a common "culture" integral to their "identity" and to focus on it as a disappearing commodity in need of revival and preservation. To this end, they set about "the rejuvenation of cultural activities." Their first project was the revival of "a long dormant festival," the Festa di San Pedro. According to Sta. Maria:

> The entire district of Praya Lane had never seen such effort being consolidated and such a momentous occasion as that which was seen on the 29th June 1967. While youths toiled labourously [*sic*], the old decorated the arches. Over two hundred yards, in a parallel order, coloured bulbs were hung amidst arches and flags. The items for the day were carefully programmed to make the occasion a memorable one. There were boat races, games, competition for the decorated boats and an open air mass to bless the occasion. The night was packed with laughter as the folks danced to their favourite melody the '*Branyo.*' . . . With this maiden success, the hearts and minds of the community was instilled with the importance of reviving our Cultural heritage. Then only the realization came that '*a race without a culture, is a race without an identity.*' (B. Sta. Maria 1982, 194; emphasis in original)

In reality, it is unlikely that in this staunch fishing community there ever was a period when the feast of Saint Peter (the patron saint of fishermen) was completely—let alone "long"—dormant. In some years the celebrations were undoubtedly grander than in others, but the religious act of cleaning and blessing the boats combined with a festive *branyo* in the evening was regularly observed by the fishermen. Poetic license aside, however, the 1967 Festa di San Pedro effectively transformed an internal community celebration into a public spectacle. Soon moved to the Settlement venue, the transformed festival ultimately marked a crucial step in the development of the Portuguese Settlement as a tourist site (see Sarkissian 1999).

In addition to organizing festivals, the Portuguese Cultural Society also formed a new group under the direction of singer Noel Felix.[18] Reflective of the community-centered ideals of the society, this group was different from those that preceded it in several respects. First, it spanned the gamut of the community, with members ranging from school children to grandparents. Next, its repertoire embraced a range of genres that together constituted the Malacca Portuguese musical world: the imported dances continued to be performed (forming a "core" repertoire), but locally composed numbers with texts in Kristang and even translated American popular songs were also featured. The most significant departure from the established format, however, was a new emphasis placed on *mata kantiga,* the traditional improvised male-female song duel sung to *branyo* music. This last change had two prime functions: first, it served to unify the community, for although only a few remaining members of the older generation were skilled in the art of verbal duelling, everyone—young and old—could dance the *branyo* together. Second, it clearly demonstrated their mixed heritage, for *mata kantiga* and *branyo* are related to *dondang sayang* and *joget,* respectively, two Malay genres particularly associated with the Malacca region and widely held to be of Portuguese origin.[19]

1969: Dark Clouds

These departures—the attempt to "revive" traditions, the inclusiveness of the new dance group, and the promotion of hybrid musical genres—must be viewed against the wider national picture, for together they demonstrate Portuguese Eurasian flexibility and ability to adapt quickly to political exigencies. By mid-1968, interethnic tension across the nation had peaked in reaction to the government's policy of special privileges for ethnic Malays. As the 1969 federal election approached, new political parties appeared on the scene, campaigning on platforms of ethnic equality and cultural pluralism. Highly emotional surface issues of education and language concealed an underlying concern about the role of individual ethnic groups in the new nation. By the time the votes were counted, the opposition parties had together won enough seats to change the balance of power. Celebrations, which began on May 13, 1969, rapidly degenerated into four days of racial riots in the streets of Kuala Lumpur. Though the riots were quickly contained, further incidents of violence—mostly perpetrated by militant Malays on what they considered an inward-looking Chinese community—persisted for another two months.

The instability preceding and savage violence following the general election sensitized the whole nation to issues of ethnic identity and to the potential fragility of their society. No one—least of all members of minority groups—wanted to be singled out. In the midst of this national crisis, local public criticism of the Portuguese Eurasian community came to a head as Malacca's chief minister, Dato' Haji Talib bin Karim, joined the debate and issued a stern warning, advising residents of the Portuguese Settlement "that they had to change their attitudes in life if they wanted to progress as true Malaysian citizens. . . . [They] should not remain in isolation but should come forward and join with the other races to take part in various development projects being implemented by the government" (*MM,* December 29, 1968).

Conscious of the prevailing national tensions and influenced by Bernard Sta. Maria's political acumen, the newly formed Portuguese Cultural Society attempted to highlight elements of their culture most compatible with the culture of ethnic Malays. The Upper Tens had used Portuguese music and dance to demonstrate their non-British identity. Now what was needed was an ability to blend in, to show that they were good Malaysians of long standing. To this end, a number of large-scale productions were staged in prestigious public venues in Malacca, Kuala Lumpur, and Singapore. In addition to the usual repertoire, new emphasis was placed on the performance of the local hybrid genres, *mata kantiga* and *branyo.* Even clothing was used to emphasize their natural hybridity:

> [One] attraction will be the "branyo," a dance similar to the ronggeng introduced in 1511 when the Portuguese conquered Malacca. . . . Teenage girls in batik with the boys using the telok balanga will give this dance a Malaysian touch. . . . The mata-kantiga (killing of words) by Mr. Noel Felix and Mrs. Rosil de Costa will give pantun lovers a chance to listen to the Portuguese version of it. (*MM,* December 6, 1968)

The strategy was successful in some quarters, at least, for the *Straits Times* review of "perhaps the world's most remarkable example of cultural survival" highlighted the key themes of longevity, survival, and hybridity: "For nearly 500 years the Portuguese Eurasian community here has clung to its religion, to many customs and to its locally evolved language to become an intriguing facet of Malaysian life" (*ST,* December 9, 1968).

Smoothing Troubled Waters

Over the next few years, media coverage of Portuguese Cultural Society productions continued to build on these stereotypic narrative threads and to echo the community's belief that music and dance were an invaluable means of generating social cohesion and maintaining solidarity. In addition to being portrayed as hardy survivors, the older members of the troupe were seen as the epitome of happy-go-lucky, singing, dancing villagers:

> A 71-year-old woman singer, Madam Rosil de Costa, a member of the 34 dancers of the Portuguese Cultural Society, believes that dancing and singing is a tonic for longevity. . . . Madam Rosil, dressed in sarong and Kebaya, said "Most of the members of the Portuguese Eurasian community in Ma-

lacca like to dance and sing as this is part of our life. Dancing and singing keep us young and happy." (*Singapore Herald,* April 12, 1971)

Although the Cultural Society's attempt to emphasize the connection between local Portuguese and Malay musical traditions must be seen primarily as a pragmatic response to a particular political climate, as a long-term strategy it was ultimately doomed to failure, for the improvisation of *mata kantiga* texts was a dying art. Rosil de Costa, the last female singer to perform in public, was also one of the last of the pre-Settlement era musicians from the ethnically mixed Praya Lane *kampung.* When she died, *mata kantiga* as an extempore male-female duelling art also died. But the *branyo* dance was far too popular to die out completely. Instead— as we shall see below—with texts and tunes transformed, it is still the most popular dance in the Portuguese Settlement.

As Bernard Sta. Maria became more involved in local politics and the land issue, he spent less time promoting the Portuguese Cultural Society, which gradually became less active. The sixty-five-member troupe gave its final large-scale performance at the Dewan Bahasa dan Pustaka in December 1975. By this time media romanticization of the community and its performing tradition was so well-established that the entire package—imported as well as local repertoire—was considered to be "carefully preserved Portuguese culture handed down to them by their ancestors, who conquered Malacca in 1511" (*Parade,* January 4, 1976).

Performing for a Living

As Cultural Society interests diverged, a smaller dance group emerged under the direction of Noel Felix. By 1972, the group—removed from Praya Lane and relocated in the Portuguese Settlement—was performing under a new name, Tropa de Malaca. By the mid-1970s, national tension had subsided and the overt demonstration of homogeneous Malaysian identity was no longer needed. Although opportunities to stage large-scale productions were now few and far between, the first stirrings of mass tourism meant that there were increasing possibilities for smaller groups. Consequently, two other groups were formed around this time: Tropa de Assunta (in 1975), based at Praya Lane and led by Stephen Theseira, and Rancho Folclorico San Pedro, based in the Portuguese Settlement.

Rancho Folclorico San Pedro was founded in 1974 by a new Portuguese priest, Fr. Augusto Sendim, who persuaded three experienced dancers and musicians—Joe Lazaroo, Walter Sequerah, and Patrick de Silva— to come out of retirement and teach the new generation of Settlement youngsters. The new group also marked the return of Christie Rodrigues to active involvement with the Malacca dance groups. Over the next decade, she and Fr. Sendim visited Portugal several times, collecting new repertoire (songs and dances) to teach their group (CRK, March 19, 1991). Right from the start, Rancho Folclorico San Pedro was different from the other groups, distinguished by a vitality and virtuosity generated by their newer repertoire.

The groups continued to perform on an irregular basis until two external developments occurred in the early 1980s. First, in 1983 the Malacca state government identified tourism as a major growth industry and began to advertise the city as "Malaysia's Historic City" (LCB, May 30, 1991). Second, a year later, the federal government allowed Eurasians of Portuguese descent to invest in Amanah Saham Nasional, a savings bond scheme otherwise open only to ethnic Malays or *bumiputras* (Malay: "sons of the soil"). The impact of tourism on the city has generated a rapid expansion of commercial opportunities for the performing groups. As their fame has increased, they have traveled all over West Malaysia and further afield to Sabah and Sarawak (East Malaysia) and to Macau. In return, groups from Macau and Portugal have visited the Settlement. While there is not enough money in cultural performance to support full-time troupes, performing has become a lucrative side income for a large number of Settlement musicians and dancers.

Three

LIVING TRADITION/
TRADITION FOR A LIVING

January 1991 If you happen to stroll along D'Albuquerque Road on a weekday evening sometime around 7:30, you might notice a group of teenagers nonchalantly hanging around No. 9. The house is hard to miss; it's the tallest one on the main street, the only one in the Settlement with a Malay-style raised porch. This particular evening the scene is typical: Joe Lazaroo leans against his wire fence, chatting to passersby and feigning disinterest in the comings and goings around him. An old man, also called Joe Lazaroo but no relation, arrives carrying a white plastic bag that conceals a tambourine. He sits on a low concrete block at the base of the porch, waiting, and pays his respects to a tiny old lady seated opposite. She is the mother of Noel Felix, leader of a rival group, but no one seems to mind her presence. Dressed in *sarong* and *kebaya* and barely able to walk, she shuffles from the far end of the Settlement each day to watch the practice. Joe looks around, wondering whether to bother fetching his guitar or simply to use the cassette Fr. Sendim left. Just at that moment, he spots Francis de Costa from No. 13, slinging a guitar over his shoulder and lighting a cigarette as he hurries to join them, late as always. Joe opts for live music, shouts for someone to bring his guitar, and watches as Francis, or "Inspector Sub" as he is known (though no one remembers quite why), goes through the familiar act of shimmying through Joe's gate without letting Chivas, the dog, escape.

Someone, probably Joe's wife Catherine, switches on the porch light, the signal that practice is about to begin. Basil Bournaparte, a rotund man with thick spectacles, emerges from the house. In one hand he has a large bass drum; in the other, he carries Joe's black guitar, the one with the mother-of-pearl inlay. The dancers   *67* line up against the wire fence in the far corner of the yard. Sub looks around, makes sure everyone is ready, then counts "two, three, four," and Joe begins to sing, "Ao nos' Algarve / do ceu azul. . . ." For an instant Joe looks out into the distance, perhaps imagining the blue Algarve sky. The dreamy look is quickly replaced by a critical eye trained on the dancers, who in their everyday clothes trot through their paces as they have done a hundred times before. They know the tune and they know their steps: the words and the faraway world they evoke barely register. Their run-though seems perfect, though Joe always spots a mistake—someone slightly late finishing a turn or a line that is not quite straight—and shouts at the perpetrator. Occasionally one of the dancers takes offense and there is an argument or (more likely) an unspoken tension in the air, but most of the time, it's water off a duck's back: they laugh, shrug their shoulders, and make sure they don't get caught again. And anyway, Joe reminds them, his shouting is nothing compared to that of Clement de Silva when he was their age.

Next it's the turn of the novice dancers. There are always youngsters wanting to join the group. Those still too small sit outside the wire fence on their bicycles and watch, subconsciously memorizing the steps as they dream of becoming glamorous dancers in their turn. Those already in the training group know it's not as easy as it looked from the other side of the fence. Joe's daughter Elaine patiently counts the beats to guide them, pulling a boy this way, pushing a girl that way. The other senior dancers sit in a huddle under the porch, relaxing and chatting as they watch the youngsters, who will gradually dance beside and eventually replace them, repeating a pattern over and over till they get it right. That, after all, was how they learned.

As usual, there are the regular spectators on the other side of the fence. Sam Hendricks from No. 8: he's only three, but knows when the dancers make mistakes. Or Carrieanne de Costa from No. 12: she has just turned one and can already hum her favorite waltz. Both her parents perform with Noel Felix's group and three of her grandparents belonged to the first Settlement group. Then there are the neighbors who watch from their yards, some nostalgically remembering the old days when they, too, were dancers. Other residents stop for a while to watch, greeting friends as they take their evening stroll. About the only people missing are the *Ropiano*s, as tourists are generically called. For most of them the Settlement is too far from the lure of Malacca Raya. Built on reclaimed land and overflowing with bars, discos, and restaurants, the neon-lit new town exudes night-time action. Only the hardiest travelers prefer this backwater on week nights. They pass by No. 9, pause for a few seconds, and walk on. They rarely take photographs, for without the lights and costumes, there's no magic.

● ● ●

This is the everyday face of music and dance in the Settlement-as-housing-estate: neither the glamorous world imagined by Settlement children nor the "authentic experience" sought by tourists. Instead it is a cottage industry for which Settlement residents are famous in the same way that they are famous for making *belachan* (dried shrimp paste) and *achar* (pickle). Like any livelihood, mastery requires skill, professionalism, and diligent practice (see fig. 9). But once again, real and imagined worlds converge, conveniently smoothing over the inherent paradox: it is and is not their tradition.

As the previous chapters suggest, the paradox is complex. The Portuguese roots of the community are defined more by ascription and accretion

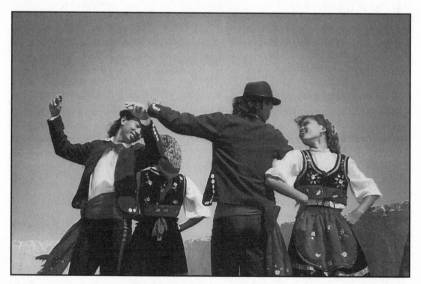

Figure 9   Rancho Folclorico San Pedro dancers, September 1990. Photograph by M. Veera Pandiyan

than necessarily by genetics. The community has carved out an identity by borrowing someone else's novelty and gradually transforming it into a "tradition," the individual elements of which have been drawn from different times and places according to the needs of the moment. The end product (now known simply as "Portuguese dance" or "cultural dance") transcends its heterogeneous origins and becomes—like the direct blood link—another bridge connecting the present with the past. When the performers put on their costumes, "they wrap themselves in a set of associations linking their music [and dance] to an idealized view of a bucolic past" (Feintuch 1993, 185). When they step onto a stage, the imaginary world of the Settlement-as-historical-monument is evoked and they are transformed into D'Albuquerque's heirs. In the glare of the spotlights, there is seepage between worlds: the musicians and dancers who perform tradition for a living become part of a living tradition.

And yet at the same time, it is not "their" tradition. It is not spontaneously performed by a broad cross-section of community members for their own enjoyment, but deliberately staged by a limited number of specially trained young people for the entertainment of outsiders. At the peak of Malacca's tourist boom (1990–92), there were five competing groups: Tropa de Malaca, Rancho Folclorico San Pedro, Tropa de Assunta, D'Tiru-Tiru Portuguese Cultural Group, and Strela di Melaka. Yet the total number of participants (including trainees and occasional performers) never exceeded about seventy-five musicians and dancers, roughly six or seven percent of the total Settlement population. Furthermore, a comparison of the various groups shows that, despite surface similarities (e.g., in costumes, core repertoire, and stereotypical movements), what appears typical is essentially unique. Each group is different, with its own history, social structure, and underlying philosophy forged by the personality of its leader. The phenomenon that residents have come to describe as their "tradition" is thus defined by and dependent on a steadily diminishing number of extraordinary individuals, who are in turn embedded in and affected by wider Settlement politics complicated by their own personal quarrels (euphemistically called "misunderstandings").

The proliferation of dance groups between 1990 and 1992 had as much to do with internal Settlement politics as with the tourism boom sweeping the nation.[1] The first "Visit Malaysia Year" (1990) certainly provided increased opportunities to perform, opportunities enhanced by the determination of Malacca's chief minister, Rahim Tamby Chik, to turn the city into a major tourist destination. Astute manipulation of the Settlement-as-historical-monument, a cornerstone of Rahim's "Historic

Malacca" package, by a visionary *Regedor* might have reinforced corporate cultural identity, provided new forms of employment, and ultimately spared the Settlement from the threat of development. The cottage industry might have become an organized business, with several performing units under the administration of a single director systematically cornering the market. Instead, long-standing disputes, conflicting egos, and consistent manipulation of volatile tempers (called "instigating") produced competing groups, each determined to outdo the others.

Getting Started

The oldest dance groups, Tropa de Malaca and Rancho Folclorico San Pedro, have been introduced already. The former, led by Noel Felix, began life as a part of Bernard Sta. Maria's Portuguese Cultural Society in 1967 and became independent in 1972; the latter, led by Joe Lazaroo, was founded by the late Fr. Sendim in 1974. Tropa de Assunta was formed a year later in response to conflict between the Settlement and Praya Lane communities. Tired of friction with youths from the Settlement, a group of Praya Lane musicians and dancers, most of whom were cousins, persuaded their family patriarch Stephen Theseira (a former member of the Portuguese Cultural Society who had often partnered Rosil de Costa in *mata kantiga* song duels) to be their leader. As a family organization based outside the Settlement, Tropa de Assunta was, from its inception, an anomaly among the dance groups.

The three groups coexisted relatively amicably until a marked increase in performing opportunities arose, due to the nationwide growth of tourism and to government promotion of the cultural show as an acceptable marker of national diversity. The development of the Settlement-as-tourist-attraction led to a corresponding increase in commercialization. Predictably, commercialization led to competition and eventually to conflict. The hunt for outside contracts and bigger fees, for example, produced increased rivalry among the groups, resulting in accusations of undercutting, sabotaging, or even stealing contracts. Money became a source of friction within groups, too, as dissatisfied members periodically accused their leaders of fiscal irregularities. Most of the time such arguments led to minor realignments: a musician or dancer might move from one group to another or even give up performing altogether.

Irreconcilable differences occasionally lead to fission. Crises, when they do occur, are usually precipitated by arrangements surrounding the annual Festa di San Pedro. Commercial success has transformed this festival from a community religious celebration—a rite of incorporation—into a nationally recognized folkloric festival.[2] As opportunities to make money (whether from winning prizes, running food and game stalls, or performing for the crowds) have proliferated, the Festa has become an annually contested battleground upon which new feuds are fought and old grievances rekindled as everyone tries to make some quick money. Underlying tensions, which simmer all year, are ignited by festival preparations and blaze in the oxygen of publicity. It no longer matters who organizes the festival or how widely they make their accounts available afterward: each year they will be accused of rigging contests, pocketing sponsorship money, and robbing the fishermen. Musicians and dancers—like practically everyone else in the Settlement—are embroiled in internal political squabbles, which are in turn enlivened by long-standing personality conflicts. On two occasions particularly intense disputes resulted in the formation of new groups: D'Tiru-Tiru Portuguese Cultural Group formed by Freddie Scully in 1985 and Strela di Melaka ("Stars of Malacca") in 1991.[3]

Practicing

Since Portuguese dance is a vocation rather than common practice, training is important. Significant differences between the groups are illuminated (and reinforced) not only in their varying attitudes towards practice but also in the demarcation of rehearsal time and space. In these terms, Rancho Folclorico San Pedro is the most visible of all the groups. Its practices are held in a public venue—Joe Lazaroo's front yard, No. 9 on the Settlement's main street, D'Albuquerque Road—at the most sociable time of day (weekday evenings), weather and enthusiasm permitting (map 2, *a*). In effect, the group issues a challenge: anyone can watch them practice—fellow residents, visitors, passing tourists, or even dancers from rival groups—for there is nothing to hide. Most of the time, the senior dancers run straight through the dances in their repertory. Individual steps and patterns are only worked on when there are new dancers to be trained. Choreography is passed from dancer to dancer and is never consciously changed. This surface transparency, however, disguises deeper workings. Repeating the same dances at each practice creates a canon; the fixity of their choreography creates an illusion of "authenticity"; and the passing of choreography from one dancer's body to the next makes it appear unchanging and "traditional."

Tropa de Malaca's practices—when they occur—are held in the backyard of the kindergarten midway along D'Aranjo Road behind the Portuguese Square (*c* in map 2). It is a semipublic venue: open enough that anyone who so desires can watch through the wire fence, yet far enough from the main street that few outsiders hear the music. The regular audience comprises women from the houses opposite the schoolyard (who often set out chairs to watch practices as they catch up on the day's news) and small children. Since Tropa de Malaca dancers are somewhat older than those of other groups and have performed together for so long, practices are only deemed necessary either for the relatively rare occasions when new musicians or dancers are admitted to the group or when senior dancers decide to reset the choreography. Musical accompaniment at practices is generally minimal, often with only Gerard de Costa (a former dancer turned singer/musician) on guitar. The dancers prefer this arrangement since they get more work done. If Noel Felix attends the practice, he usually runs through pieces from top to bottom, without stopping to iron out problems. Like Joe Lazaroo, Noel believes that there is a right ("traditional") way and a wrong way to perform a particular dance. When he is not there, however, the dancers experiment with new choreographic "variations," and each member is encouraged to request any dance or section of a dance that he or she may find difficult.[4]

D'Tiru-Tiru's practices are held each Monday and Thursday from 8:30 till 10 P.M. in the backyard of Freddie Scully's house at No. 21 Eredia Road (*b* in map 2). It is a semiprivate venue, located on the periphery of the more affluent east side of the Settlement, well away from public areas. Few residents have cause to wander that far down Eredia Road; there are only a few houses beyond Scully's and a dead end in the road. Even if a curious onlooker wanted to investigate, nothing would be visible, since the yard is enclosed by a high wooden fence. Despite their apparent invisibility, D'Tiru-Tiru's practices can be heard all over the Settlement, for it is the only group that regularly uses amplification. As activity winds down for the day, the amplified sounds of Scully's voice and D'Tiru-Tiru's musicians are broadcast on the still night air. Behind the fence, D'Tiru-Tiru functions much like a youth club, perhaps a reminder of the days gone by when Scully was young and organized the first Portuguese Settlement Youth Club. Rehearsals double as social gatherings: members hang out at Freddie's house before and after practice, and there is always a short break during which soft drinks are served and the youngsters are given an opportunity to relax, chat, and, in some cases, flirt. The boys, in particular, compete for attention by showing off their latest hip-hop dance routines

Map 2
The Portuguese Settlement,
1991.

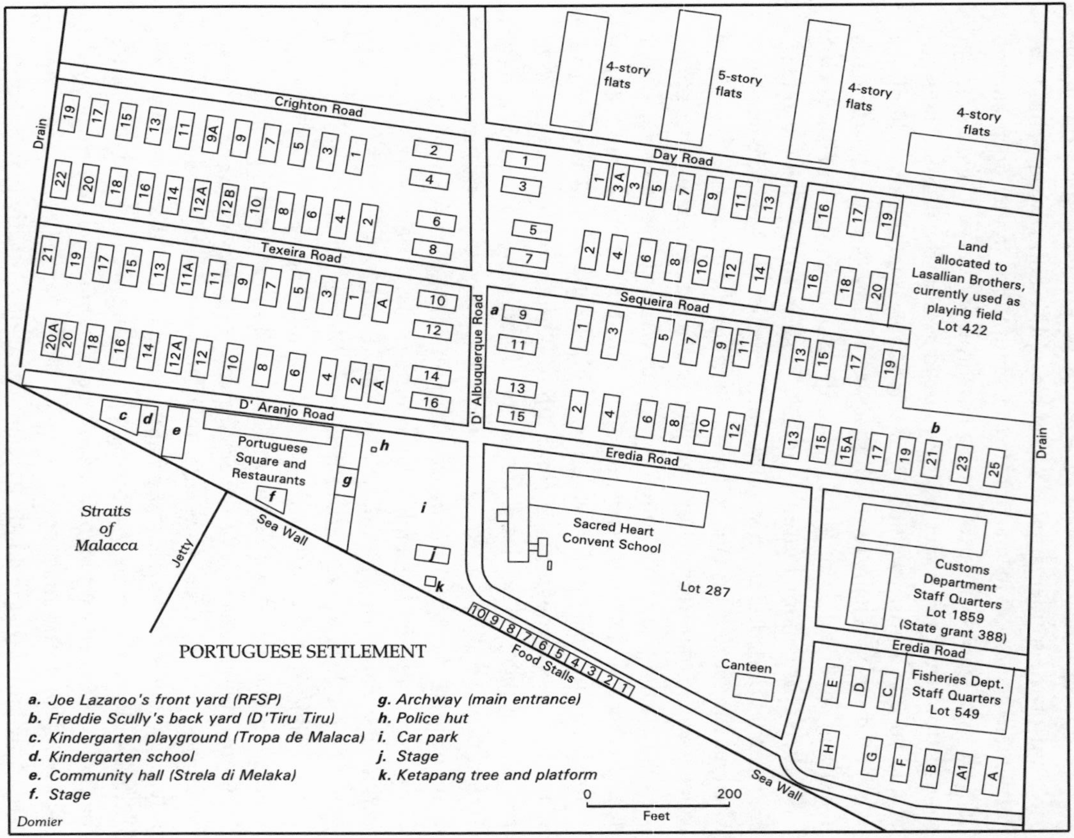

PORTUGUESE SETTLEMENT

a. Joe Lazaroo's front yard (RFSP)
b. Freddie Scully's back yard (D'Tiru Tiru)
c. Kindergarten playground (Tropa de Malaca)
d. Kindergarten school
e. Community hall (Strela di Melaka)
f. Stage

g. Archway (main entrance)
h. Police hut
i. Car park
j. Stage
k. Ketapang tree and platform

Domier

accompanied by Georgie de Costa's son, Leo, on synthesizer. Scully—in his day the Settlement rock-and-roll king—indulgently encourages the dancers, sometimes even offering suggestions. In the competitive world of the Portuguese Settlement, D'Tiru-Tiru's partial secrecy is interpreted as proof that the group has something to hide. Accusations that Scully and de Costa "stole" dances from the other groups (particularly from de Costa's former group, Tropa de Malaca) are countered by D'Tiru-Tiru's claims to preeminent "authenticity" traced directly to the minister's visit. Georgie de Costa, one of the three Settlement boys who sang at the 1952 Tea Entertainment (see fig. 6, above in chap. 2), was (until his death in 1994) the last active member of the original Settlement group.

Strela di Melaka, the shortest-lived group, practiced in the small hall attached to the Portuguese Square (*e* in map 2). Although the location was adjacent to Tropa de Malaca's practice space at the kindergarten, rehearsals could neither be seen nor heard. The hall's opaque slatted windows were always closed; onlookers of any sort were discouraged by "guards" who patrolled the exterior; and practices were scheduled at different times and days of the week. The secrecy was deliberate: Strela di Melaka had not only copied dances (primarily from Tropa de Malaca) but also lured dancers from all three groups with financial incentives. Until their first public performance, few Settlement residents knew the identity of Strela di Melaka performers.

Having by far the smallest pool of musicians and dancers, the Praya Lane community's Tropa de Assunta performs irregularly and practices even less. With no substitute dancers to cover members who are not available, they often turn down regular engagements in favor of special (usually higher-paying) one-time functions. As a family concern (most of the members are Stephen Theseira's adult children and their cousins), organization and financial arrangements are informal.

Group Organization

Group organization spans the gamut from highly authoritarian to extremely easygoing. Joe Lazaroo and Freddie Scully are both strong leaders who dominate their groups and control all domains, practical (from arranging performances to paying performers) and artistic (from selecting to training musicians and dancers). Scully is somewhat less authoritarian than Lazaroo: he often asks his senior musicians[5] and dancers for their input in decision making, and even his youngest dancers treat him as a strict but benevolent uncle. More easygoing as leaders, Noel Felix and

Stephen Theseira both allow group participation in decision making and may even turn practical and artistic responsibilities over to younger members. In Theseira's case, the family nature of his group has made such delegation easier.

Rancho Folclorico San Pedro and Tropa de Malaca provide the clearest contrast between the groups. Joe Lazaroo acts as sole manager for Rancho Folclorico San Pedro. He is responsible for all the contracts and for arranging transportation to and from shows. His wife, Catherine, usually travels with the group as chaperone, dresser, and makeup artist. Discipline is strict, particularly when the group is performing out of town. On these occasions Joe takes his position in loco parentis seriously; anyone caught disobeying his rules is sent home. Tropa de Malaca, in contrast, is more communally oriented. The dancers are, on average, older than those performing with the other groups; some are married with children. Several members have been with the group since Noel Felix brought it to the Settlement in 1972. As one might expect with such longevity, camaraderie is strong—not only among the dancers but between musicians and dancers. The pervading atmosphere is lighthearted and informal; newer members say they joined because, unlike the other groups, "it's not very strict and you can joke around." Noel's laissez faire attitude and willingness to delegate authority have created a democratic organization in which each member of the group has a voice in decision making.[6] Gerard Lazaroo, still dancing in his early forties, acts as manager, soliciting contracts and arranging logistics, but before accepting a major contract, he always calls a group meeting to discuss acceptance and availability of dancers. Since hotel contracts usually specify a fixed number of musicians and dancers, members usually divide the time: those who are unemployed may perform for the duration while others go for a few days and are substituted. This way the entire group shares the experience and no one misses too much work or school.

Financial Organization

Handling of finances also varies from group to group. More authoritarian leaders like Lazaroo and Scully control finances tightly but have formal accounting systems so that malcontents have no cause to accuse them of fiscal irregularities. Characteristically, Strela di Melaka's financial dealings were secretive, although rumors abounded that (unlike any of the other groups) dancers were offered financial rewards to join and additional stipends for attending practice, while musicians were offered double the amount paid to dancers. The two more democratic groups, Tropa de Malaca and Tropa de Assunta, both maintain less formal financial arrangements. While no one can earn a living from Portuguese dance alone, it is a useful supplement to regular employment for musicians and older dancers and the main source of pocket money for youngsters, who often contribute part of their earnings to the general family income.

As might be expected, Rancho Folclorico San Pedro has a more formal system of accounting. Each member of the group, including Catherine Lazaroo, receives an equal share of the fee once transportation and miscellaneous extra expenses have been deducted. In addition, Joe takes an extra share to cover his expenses (telephone calls, electricity, etc.) and puts the remaining money aside into a central fund for running costs (e.g., costumes, guitar strings, special dinners or gifts, etc.) and for rewarding educational achievements. Small cash bonuses are given to dancers who pass their Form 3 or Form 5 examinations. To prove they have received their share, members sign a ledger when collecting their money: cash payments are made as soon as a check has been banked and cleared. The accounts are never formally audited, but each member has the right (though few have the temerity or the ability) to inspect them. As the most prominent group, Rancho Folclorico San Pedro is occasionally awarded large sums by the government or by foundations in Macau. Such windfalls are usually applied to the purchase of new instruments or sets of costumes.

With career experience as a finance clerk, Freddie Scully created a complex yet highly flexible accounting system for D'Tiru-Tiru. It functions somewhat like a bank, allowing maximum individual choice. Each member is allocated an "account" in Scully's master ledger. As he or she performs, earnings are recorded in the ledger. Depending on personal need, a member can choose to withdraw cash as it is earned, withdraw small sums for pocket money and save the balance, or even save everything and withdraw a lump sum at a later date. (Georgie de Costa and his two children, for example, pooled their combined earnings and withdrew a lump sum once a year before Christmas.) A portion of each fee is set aside for running costs, costumes, equipment, and educational needs; school children may be given bonuses to help pay examination fees, purchase textbooks, or as rewards for passing exams. The size of the portion allocated to the central fund depends on the size of the fee: if a fee is unusually large, Freddie sets a proportionately larger sum aside rather than "spoil" the dancers by giving them too much. Although Scully's intention is to teach his youngsters a lesson about managing their own money, his banking system has resulted in a greater emphasis placed on financial gain. Even the tiniest dancers in his junior group argue over money, complaining that they get a smaller percentage than older dancers (who, of course, perform the lion's share of any given program).

Tropa de Malaca's financial arrangements are the least formal. Gerard Lazaroo banks the checks and pays everyone cash when the money has cleared; there is no book to sign. Each group member receives an equal share and an unspecified percentage is put into a central fund for costumes, guitar strings, dinners, occasional birthday presents or parties, and other miscellaneous expenses. No special incentives are offered for academic achievement as few members are of school age. Everyone in the group trusts Gerard, though from time to time a jealous member or an interfering relative will try to cause trouble by questioning his honesty.

Leaders

The dependence of the cultural groups on a diminishing number of central figures or "stars" is emphasized by the sharp decline in the number of independent groups since 1992. Strela di Melaka, for example, never stood a chance of becoming established because it had no such leader. George Alcantra, while politically powerful, could not hold the group together because he was not a musician. He tried to hire others (including Noel Felix) to perform for him, but wage laborers had no vested interest in becoming leaders and there were not enough leaders to go around. Though Noel and a few of his regular musicians played with Strela di Melaka for the 1991 Festa di San Pedro celebrations, outraged protests from the rest of Tropa de Malaca speedily terminated their moonlighting. Without live music, Strela di Melaka could not compete for outside contracts and, before long, the group was disbanded. Tropa de Assunta, the Praya Lane group, also faded out by the mid-1990s. Leader Stephen Theseira, suffering from poor health, turned the group over to his adult children, who continued for a while until lack of recruits forced them to disband.

The most dramatic reversal of fortune, however, was experienced by D'Tiru-Tiru, the healthiest of all the groups in 1992. Freddy Scully was never a good singer; it was always his talent as emcee, organizer, and canny impresario that held his group together. For example, in 1991, after several senior boys left for Singapore in search of work, he decided to plan for the future on a large scale. Unlike Felix and Lazaroo (who trained a few replacement dancers at a time, slowly integrating them into the main group), Scully began to train a set of much younger dancers in the seven-to ten-year-old range. His showman's hunch soon paid off: by 1992, the diminutive dancers of his junior group were captivating tourists in public on the Portuguese Settlement stage. Yet despite the group's vitality and promise for the future, it did not survive Freddie Scully's sudden death in March 1994. D'Tiru-Tiru was disbanded because no one—not even Georgie de Costa, who himself passed away a few weeks later, or Scully and de Costa's children, several of whom had worked with their fathers as musicians, dancers, and teachers—could replace him as leader.

By 1996 two groups remained—Rancho Folclorico San Pedro and Tropa de Malaca. The entire performing tradition for which the Settlement is famous, the culture the headman urges the youngsters to maintain, is now defined by two men: Joe Lazaroo and Noel Felix. These two men, who are far from typical, have come to embody what people *believe* their tradition to be. Despite their uniqueness (perhaps even because of it), Lazaroo and Felix have come to be considered—like Feintuch's 1920s Northumbrian piper, Tom Clough—"the best model of the tradition" (Feintuch 1993, 198). And yet, as the following comparison demonstrates, Lazaroo and Felix are unlike each other in almost every respect.

Joe Lazaroo

Emmanuel Bosco Lazaroo (b. 1941), nicknamed "Joe," is easily the most famous resident of the Portuguese Settlement. The subject of a Malaysian airline in-flight magazine feature, "Say Hello, Joe" (Stier 1990), Joe has achieved a status otherwise reserved for monuments: tour buses pause in front of his house. Special visitors to the Settlement, especially those from Portugal or Macau, invariably end up on Joe's porch, drinking whisky and nostalgically singing *fados* to the accompaniment of his guitar. Significantly, though Joe was born and raised in the Settlement, he is not the stereotypical happy-go-lucky poor fisherman. His ancestors were neither "poor fisherfolk" nor former Upper Tens. In fact, as grandson of first *Regedor* Felix Danker, and eldest son of former Settlement secretary George Bosco Lazaroo, he is probably as close to Settlement aristocracy as one can get. He has spent all his life in Malacca, married a Nonya wife, and has two children, Edmund (b. 1970) and Elaine (b. 1975), both of whom perform with his dance group. He lived outside the Settlement for a few years after getting married, but moved back after inheriting his grandfather's house. Until he retired in 1996, Joe worked for the Public Works Department (Malay: Jabatan Kerja Raya) as supervisor of a road-building crew. Not content with retirement, Joe and his wife started a restaurant in the Portuguese Square in September 1997. Nowadays, Joe can usually be found in the evenings with a big smile on his face, behind his own bar at Papa Joe's:

> He comes on strong introducing himself by paraphrasing a classic Johnny Cash song. "How do you do? I'm Joe Lazaroo, and I am going to kill you." Then he dissipates this apparent threat with an infectious, twinkle-eyed smile and a ready hand, thrust out for you to shake. . . . There's no doubt about it: Joe has charisma. I was watching him sing one night, not one of his regular performances but, rather, a cameo he was doing because he just can't resist a microphone. His happy tenor voice poured out over the audience. . . . His eyes closed as he relished a particular note and the woman next to me commented, "His eyes twinkle even when he closes them." (Stier 1990, 35, 36)

Joe has been involved with Portuguese dance almost since its inception. He was present at the 1952 Tea Entertainment and was, in fact, the only Settlement resident officially listed on the program. Slightly too young to be part of the first Settlement group, he joined Clement de Silva's group by the late 1950s, where he came to know Clement's sister-in-law, Christie Rodrigues, and was an instructor of Freddie Scully's Portuguese Settlement Youth Club group in the 1960s. When Fr. Sendim and Christie Rodrigues founded Rancho Folclorico San Pedro in 1974, Joe was the obvious choice as leader. Like many born stars, he dominates by force of personality (fig. 10).[7] Star quality aside, Joe is a consummate professional. Although he speaks and sings in Kristang, Joe is linguistically English dominant. He works hard at his craft: he keeps typed copies of all his lyrics, compiles documentary packets about his group, and makes an effort to learn new Portuguese songs from visitors and recordings. He performs Portuguese dance for a living—not only for himself, but to enhance the lives of those around him. He is proud that he has given several generations of Settlement youngsters the chance to travel, to fly, to stay in first-class hotels, and to shake hands with dignitaries. He measures his success in the way fees have increased over the last few years.[8] He will not tell you that he enjoys the public attention, too, but it is obvious that he does: he is a gregarious man and loves being a celebrity.

Noel Felix

Noel Felix (b. 1932) is about as different from Joe Lazaroo as night is from day. To begin with, unlike Joe, he is linguistically Kristang dominant and does fit the "poor fisherfolk" stereotype. His family, originally from Praya Lane, moved to the Settlement and settled at the far end of Texeira

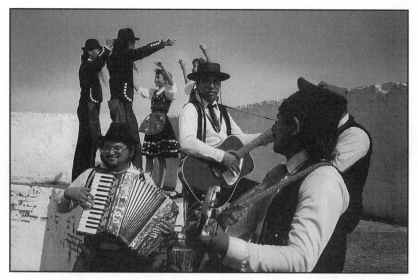

Figure 10 Joe Lazaroo *(center with black guitar)* and Rancho Folclorico San Pedro, September 1990. Photograph by M. Veera Pandiyan

Road in one of the houses built by the British government. Having had virtually no schooling, Noel started fishing with his father at the age of seven. Illiterate and with no job prospects apart from fishing, Noel joined the British army in 1952 at the age of nineteen. His ability as a singer was soon noticed, and he became popular with the British officers, one of whom taught him to read and write. Army Talent Time competitions provided his first experience of public performance. Demobbed in 1958, Noel returned to Malacca and joined the water company (Malay: Lembaga Air Melaka), where he remained until he retired at the age of 55. He married within the community and has four children, three daughters and one son, and several grandchildren. Only his oldest adopted daughter, Connie, became a dancer (though many of his nephews and nieces have followed in her footsteps). None of his three biological children have shown any interest in music or dance.[9] Noel supplemented his government pension by fishing part-time (until poor health forced him to give up in the early 1990s) and performing with Tropa de Malaca.

Stationed away from Malacca for much of the 1950s, Noel was not present for the Portuguese minister's visit nor did he belong to Clement de Silva's early group. Instead, he learned the repertoire by rote directly from Arthur Sta. Maria. When forming his Portuguese Cultural Society, Bernard Sta. Maria chose Noel as one of the leaders because of his reputa-

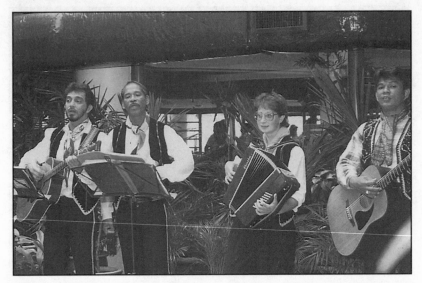

Figure 11   Noel Felix and musicians (*left to right:* Edward Nunis, Noel Felix, author, Jerry Perera), September 1990.

tion as a singer and composer. He was also one of the few remaining *mata kantiga* singers, able not only to improvise *mata kantiga* quatrains in Kristang but also to *pantun*—to improvise—*dondang sayang* quatrains in Malay. In his younger days, Noel had even entered *dondang sayang* competitions and battled against Malay and Baba singers. Bernard's intention was not simply to perform the imported Portuguese dance repertoire but to preserve *branyo* and *mata kantiga,* the traditional hybrid music of the mixed-race community. Noel Felix was a last link with the duelling tradition, as was another member of the Portuguese Cultural Society group, Stephen Theseira. Both partnered the last female *mata kantiga* dueller, Rosil de Costa.

If Joe Lazaroo has charisma, Noel Felix has presence. Not a dynamic leader on stage, he exudes none of the showmanship or sparkling patter that characterize Joe's performances. Instead he is low key—almost deadpan—in his presentation, standing a little apart from his musicians and playing nothing larger than a tambourine or a mouth organ (see fig. 11). Yet when he sings, there is an aura about him that commands attention. His easygoing good nature spills over into the group. Performances may not always be as polished as those of Joe's group, but everyone has fun and no one is scared of his temper. If someone makes an error, it is nothing to get upset about; after all, he believes the only way to learn is by making mistakes. Off stage he comes across as laconic and unhurried. While Joe might be out on his porch of an afternoon pecking away at his typewriter, dubbing tapes, or being interviewed, Noel might be out gambling under the *ketapang* tree or, more likely, at home taking a siesta.

Over the past few years, Noel has slowed down and is content to leave day-to-day running of the group to the younger generation. Although he continues to perform, his voice is no longer as strong or accurate as it once was and he tires easily. Nevertheless, he still has a well-defined sense of cultural responsibility. The man who, despite financial insecurity, turned down offers to cook at hotels or on oil rigs to remain at the helm of Tropa de Malaca says that "to be a culture man, it's not easy." Unlike Joe—who sometimes wields his group as a weapon, refusing to perform for anyone who quarrels with him—Noel performs what he sees as his cultural duty for the sake of the community and particularly, his grandchildren. Occasionally this gets him into trouble. For example, he received heavy criticism, not least from some members of his own group, in 1992 for helping Strela di Melaka. What others saw as betrayal was, in his opinion, for the greater good—to ensure there was Portuguese dance for the Festa di San Pedro. His many years of service to the community were finally acknowledged at the 1996 San Pedro festival when he was presented with a Seiko watch and certificate celebrating his lifelong cultural achievement.

The Next Generation

But what of the future? Neither Joe Lazaroo nor Noel Felix can continue forever. What will happen to the "tradition" once its two paradigmatic leaders are no longer on the scene? It is, of course, a matter for speculation, but there are encouraging signs. Both Joe and Noel are grooming successors, Edmund Lazaroo and Gerard de Costa, respectively. It is remarkable how closely Edmund and Gerard replicate the contrasting backgrounds, experience, and philosophies of their mentors.

Edmund first learned to dance with his father's group, Rancho Folclorico San Pedro. Like his father, he is not the stereotypical Portuguese Settlement resident. Educated at the University of Macau, he returned to Malacca and has a white-collar job in the nearby town of Muar. He plays guitar and sings with the group whenever his work permits; Joe has started sending him out on minor contracts as leader. There is no question that Edmund knows the dance repertory well and that he is slowly learning Joe's enormous song repertoire. Like his father, however, he performs tradition for a living. It is the only kind of music he performs and he has—so far—shown no signs of breaking away from established choreography and repertoire.

Gerard de Costa began dancing with Tropa de Malaca in his mid-teens. He has been with the group continuously ever since and has made the transition from dancer to guitarist-singer. Like Noel, he more closely resembles the stereotypical Settlement resident. His mother, her two sisters, their spouses and all their children grew up in a single—crowded—house on Texeira Road. He does not fish (though his father did so full time until relatively recently) but has a blue-collar job driving a truck for the power company, Tenaga Nasional. Although Edmund and Gerard are both second-generation dancers whose parents learned from Clement de Silva, Gerard's pedigree is slightly more "authentic" (and certainly more complex). Both his parents, Josephine (née Theseira) and Domingos de Costa, were members of the first Settlement group, as was his uncle, Georgie de Costa. Gerard emulated his parents by marrying a fellow dancer, Anne de Mello, whose father, Norman, was yet another member of the first group. All of his brothers and many of his cousins have, at one time or another, participated in Portuguese dance. In fact, between them, the De Costa, Theseira, and de Mello families can boast roughly forty-five dancers and ten musicians over three generations, spread among all the groups from the first Settlement group on down (with the exception of Tropa de Asunta).

Most significantly, like Noel (and unlike Edmund), Gerard is an all-round musician. Music is an organic part of his life, even at work. When not driving trucks for Tenaga Nasional, he is a guitarist for the Tenaga Nasional band.[10] He also keeps Tropa de Malaca going, directing rehearsals and often substituting as leader when Noel is feeling unwell. Given a freer rein than Edmund, Gerard is already creatively experimenting with new choreography for Tropa de Malaca dances. In his spare time, he plays for parties, weddings, and other functions thrown by Settlement people in Malacca and by Portuguese Eurasians as far afield as Seremban and Kuala Lumpur. He is in great demand because he is one of the few younger generation musicians able to sing *mata kantiga* verses for *branyo* dances. Never consciously studying the art, he has memorized stock verses from many sources, most particularly from singing with Noel and from his mother, Josephine de Costa.

Although there are many differences between Edmund and Gerard, the connections are striking. Roughly the same age, these two rather shy young men of very different educational and musical backgrounds have become extremely close friends in recent years. Though Gerard is the leading musician with Tropa de Malaca, he and his wife, Anne, spend much of their spare time hanging out with Edmund at Joe's house or helping out at the restaurant. Gerard even performs with Joe and Edmund when they need an extra musician for strolling engagements. As is the way of the Settlement, the friendship between the two young musicians was cemented when Edmund became the godfather of Gerard's son, Jeremy (b. 1993).[11] What this friendship will mean in the long run for the Portuguese dance phenomenon remains to be seen.

Four

FORGING A REPERTOIRE, DOMESTICATING A DIASPORA

Sunday Mail, July 3, 1977: **You must give it to them though. When it comes to bringing out the guitar and kicking off your shoes, these folks must be the most natural. It seems like they are born with music in their souls and dancing is part of their nature.**

Up stage the dancers performed beautifully to entertain the crowd with their colorful costumes—the Farapera, Anda Roda and, of course, the Branyho [*sic*]—all part of a rich culture inherited from the Portuguese. And down stage on the field the people joined in the dancing under the spotlight.

Tradition seems to run in their veins. Conscious of the fact that they are a special, if somewhat distant, part of the history of the country, in particular of Malacca, these poor but proud descendants of those seafaring Potuguese [*sic*] conquistadores (who anchored themselves in Malacca in the 15th century and plied the Straits) try hard to keep alive their heritage.

• • •

The Star, March 27, 1985: **Most of the songs can be traced back to the 16th Century, if the titles are any clue.**

Many are related to the sea, such as *Ala Marineyeros* (My Dear Soldiers [*sic*]) and *Naruda Mantiguera* (O Sailor Boy). Others are haunting love songs such as *Oh Amour* (My Love) and *Floris Yeo Kubisa* (Flower That I Admire). . . .

The folk dances run the gamut from *Riba de Barku* (Dancing On The Deck Of The Ship), *Vera Hi* (Turning Around) to the ever popular *Branyjo* [*sic*] (joget) number *Jingkli Nona.*

• • •

Newspaper reviews like these (and countless others written over the years) simultaneously illuminate and reinforce the romanticized image of the Settlement-as-historical-monument. By now the picture should be familiar: first, Settlement residents are depicted as poor but proud descendants of seafaring Portuguese conquerors, born with music and dance in their souls and tradition coursing through their veins, bravely struggling to keep their age-old heritage alive. Next—as in other successful retellings of the history of the people—the passage of time is condensed, skipping lightly between the Portuguese past (vaguely located, as in the above examples, sometime between the fifteenth and sixteenth centuries) and the Malaysian present. Finally, music and dance form a bridge that links both past with present and costumed dancers performing on stage with ordinary residents dancing off stage.

The sanctioned space of the cultural show functions as a crucible, transforming an eclectic accretion of material from all over the Portuguese world into an apparently homogenous corpus. In the glare of the spotlights, songs and dances from different times and places are serendipitously juxtaposed, fluidly linking Malacca to the Portuguese diaspora across both time and space. Old Portuguese folk dances are performed alongside newer folkloric dances imported from Portugal; locally composed songs with lyrics in Kristang are followed by "Jinkly Nona," sung in the same language but part of a nexus that stretches from Goa to Macau; and Portuguese *fado* (learned by heart, sung with conviction, but seldom fully understood) compete with local favorites, whose tunes sometimes turn out to be surprisingly familiar. The on-stage collision between real and imagined worlds is thus also a collision between domestic and diasporic worlds. On the one hand, each song and dance possesses its own history, its own series of past associations. These pasts, like shadows, are always present in performance—whether the performers are aware of them or not—and any combination of them may (or may not) be recognized by members of the audience. As James Clifford (1997, 207) has suggested of museum exhibits, songs and dances are cultural texts that cannot "be read from a stable location"; the same text can result in contradictory readings that are determined by the different life histories and experiences of the viewers. This chance element ensures that the precise configuration of the diaspora viewed on stage is effectively constructed anew in each performance. On the other hand, however, through repetition and gradual variation, the heteroglot potpourri is in the process of being transformed into a uniquely local repertoire: as the diaspora is slowly domesticated, the shadows are eclipsed. The music and dance, once imported, are becoming so deeply rooted in Settlement life that residents old enough to remember the first dance group nevertheless exhort youngsters to "keep up their culture." The younger generation see the repertoire as an homogenous, unbroken tradition stretching back to the sixteenth century.

A cursory examination of the dance tunes mentioned in the opening reviews quickly illustrates the complexity of the situation. To begin with, "Vera Hi"—anglicized here into a girl's name, but better known as "O Vira" or "O Vira Vamos"—was one of the two dances performed for the Portuguese minister's visit in 1952. Learned by upper-class Eurasians from books like Lucile Armstrong's *Dances of Portugal,* it was described therein as one of the many variations of *vira* (a type of turning dance) from the Lisbon region (Armstrong 1948, 35). "O Vira" has remained in the repertoire of all the Settlement cultural groups, although each has modified the choreography and only Rancho Folclorico San Pedro continues to play it in the original minor mode. The source for "Anda Roda" (also called "O Limao" after the first words of its chorus) is unknown, but Ida de Silva remembers learning it from notation and performing it on concert programs by about 1953 (IRS, January 1, 1991). Although no one remembers how or when "Fara Pera" was introduced, it does appear to have originated in Portugal over a century ago: its melody and text appear in Armando Leça's collection of popular Portuguese music, where the author identifies it as a *farrapeira* (a genre, not a title) from coastal Beira and adds that the same melody can be found in César das Neves's *Cancioneiro de Músicas* of 1893 (Leça ca. 1983, 126). "Riba di barku," in contrast, is not a Portuguese folk dance at all; it is one of the dances composed locally by Noel Felix for the Portuguese Cultural Society troupe in the late 1960s.

While the four songs mentioned above are equally diverse, none "can be traced back to the 16th century." "Ala Marinheiros" (a song addressed to sailors, not soldiers) was introduced by the Upper Tens in the early 1950s. Josephine de Costa, a member of the first Settlement dance group, still remembers the words she learned from Clement de Silva over forty years ago, even though she has never understood their meaning (JTC, July 1, 1991). "Naruda Mantiguera," another song from the same period, provides a salutary reminder of what can happen when unfamiliar words are absorbed into oral tradition. Confusion is clear from the outset, for the song has nothing to do with a *manteigueira,* a butter dish. The current Settlement title, "Na ruda ma figuera," is derived from the first line of the text; it has no meaning in Kristang, but is an approximation of *na roda duma fugeira,* the first line of a Portuguese song called "Ravela

Nos Namoricas" that appears in Joe Lazaroo's typescript collection of song texts. The other two songs, "Floris Yo Kubisá" and "O Amor," are both local. The former is a lyrical love song composed by Noel Felix in the late 1960s; the latter, a cowboy yodeling song with a Kristang text, owes more to local imitations of Jimmie Rodgers than to any Portuguese model and is attributed both to Norman de Mello—another member of the first Settlement dance group—and to Noel Felix.

Finally, the *branyo*—the sole item mentioned in both reviews—is the only part of the stage repertoire that is also part of ordinary Settlement life and the only dance that could unite the cultural groups with ordinary residents "down stage on the field." It is staple fare at community celebrations and the favorite dance of residents, young and old. It is uniquely theirs; yet, like them, it has a foot in both the Portuguese and Malaysian worlds. On the one hand, "Jinkly Nona" verses, collected as far apart as Goa and Macau, link the Settlement to a vast Portuguese cultural diaspora (Jackson 1990, 5–6). On the other hand, the connection between *branyo* and the Malay social dance, *joget,* has resulted in "Jinkly Nona" being considered a national folk-tune by the Malaysian general public. In fact, the connection is so close that James Chopyak (1986, 126–27) used the melody of "Jinkly Nona" as "an idealized example of a typical joget."

Scratching the Surface

Even from this small sample, then, it is clear that each song and dance brings its own complex history to the stage. In order to understand how these multiple pasts coexist and interact and how, through contemporary processes of domestication, the pasts are being erased, we must hold the entire repertoire up for careful scrutiny. In so doing, the first thing we notice is that there is not actually a single repertoire. At the broadest level, whatever the history or provenance of a given piece outside the Settlement, residents make a distinction between what they call "our music" and what they call "Portuguese music."[1] Closer examination of this indigenous taxonomy reveals that "our music" comprises two subcategories: first, songs and dances introduced during the 1950s by musically literate Upper Tens and passed on orally to subsequent generations of Settlement musicians and dancers; and second, songs and dances created by Settlement residents between 1967 and 1972, the period during which Bernard Sta. Maria's Portuguese Cultural Society was active. Music classified as "Portuguese" was introduced after 1974.

Table 1 Portuguese Dances Introduced During the 1950s ("Our Music")

Name of dance	Source (first performance)	TdeM	RFSP	TdeA	d'T-T
Anda Roda/O Limao	(known by 1953)	x	x		x
Baté Peu	Armstrong/Ribatejo "Paderinha"	x			x
Fara Pera	unknown [from Beira according to Leça]	x			x
Kamasha	uncertain (possibly mid-1950s)	x	x		x
Korradinyo	Armstrong/Beira "A Rosa"		x		
O Malhao, old version	(known by 1953)	x			x
O Vira	Armstrong/Lisbon "Vira" (1952)	x	x		x
Portuguese Washer-woman[a]	(notation found in 1956)	x			x
Regadinyo[b]	unknown/Minho	x	x		x
Ti' Anika	(known by 1953)	x	x		x
Tiru Liru Liru	Ruy Cinatti, Fr. Pintado's friend (1952)		x		x
Verdi Gayo	(known by 1953)	x			x
Vira Atra Passados	Armstrong/Minho "Vira Extrapassada"	x			x

NOTE: TdeM = Tropa de Malaca; RFSP = Rancho Folclorico San Pedro; TdeA = Tropa de Assunta (Praya Lane); and d'T-T = D'Tiru-Tiru.

a. "The Portuguese Washerwoman" (also known as "Lavadeira di Portugal" or "Madonna di Portugal") has an unusual story associated with its introduction. Ida de Silva found the sheet music around 1956 when she was accompanying a local ballet class. The ballet teacher, Mrs. David Peirce, subsequently choreographed a dance to fit the music (IRS, January 1, 1991). More of an artistic interpretation (including drunken staggering by the boys) than a folk dance, "The Portuguese Washerwoman" remains an oddity in the repertoire. Musically, too, it is exceptional, comprising several short sections repeated in irregular order with an abrupt modulation (from C major to F major) in one of the sections.

b. "Regadinyo" is often paired with "Kamasha," especially by Rancho Folclorico San Pedro, which performs the two dances as a medley. Although there is strong evidence that "Kamasha" was introduced in the 1950s, it is by no means certain that "Regadinyo" was introduced at the same time. The fact that it is performed by all three groups and has relatively straightforward choreography suggests, however, that it may be an old dance and not from the more virtuosic Sendim-Rodrigues repertoire. Furthermore, although no regional association is given, a close variant of the tune appears in an early collection of Portuguese dance (João do Rio 1909, 444–47). The Malacca version of "Regadinyo" also appears in a collection of traditional Portuguese music published in Macau, where it is defined as a melody from the Minho region (Moura 1994).

Dances

If we organize the dance repertoire according to this system of classification and indicate which group performs a given piece (see tables 1, 2, and 3),[2] we notice something else: just as the cultural groups appear homogeneous but are individual, so too are the dances they perform. While shows may superficially appear interchangeable, the fact remains that each group performs a unique combination of dances that reinforces many of

Table 2 Dances Composed by Settlement Residents, 1967 to 1972 ("Our Music")

Name of dance	Source	TdeM	RFSP	TdeA	d'T-T
Alegrá[a]	Stephen Theseira	(x)		x	
Allegros companyeros	Stephen Theseira			x	
Kapten di barku	Noel Felix	x			
Lembransa di antigu	Stephen Theseira			x	
Pasturinyu	Noel Felix	x			
Rentu di jarding	Stephen Theseira			x	
Riba di barku	Noel Felix	x			

NOTE: TdeM = Tropa de Malaca; RFSP = Rancho Folclorico San Pedro; TdeA = Tropa de Assunta (Praya Lane); and d'T-T = D'Tiru-Tiru.

a. Rather than performing Stephen Theseira's version of this song, Noel Felix uses the same melody to accompany a song he calls "El Bayo."

Table 3 Portuguese Dances Introduced After 1974 ("Portuguese Music")

Name of dance	Source	TdeM	RFSP	TdeA	d'T-T
A la viola	videotape				x
Ao nossa Algarve	Sendim-Rodrigues/Algarves region		x		
Asas brancas	Sendim-Rodrigues		x		
Baile de roda	Sendim-Rodrigues		x		
Bailinyo de Madeira	Sendim-Rodrigues/Madeira region		x		
Cana bedri	videotape				x
Minha Rosinha	Sendim-Rodrigues		x		x
O Malhao (new version)	Sendim-Rodrigues		x		
Tirana	cassette				x
Vira Cross	cassette				x
Vira di Bairu Português	Joe Lazaroo		x		
Vira d'Tiru-Tiru	videotape				x
Vira Sta. Marta	Sendim-Rodrigues/Sta. Marta da Portuzelo, Minho region		x		x

NOTE: TdeM = Tropa de Malaca; RFSP = Rancho Folclorico San Pedro; TdeA = Tropa de Assunta (Praya Lane); and d'T-T = D'Tiru-Tiru.

the differences between the groups themselves. For example, all three Settlement groups share dances from the 1950s, which I shall call "core" repertoire, but little else. Tropa de Malaca performs core dances plus those composed by its leader, Noel Felix. Rancho Folclorico San Pedro, in contrast, performs fewer core dances, none of Felix's work, and all the post-1974 pieces associated with Fr. Sendim and Christie Rodrigues. D'Tiru-Tiru, formed by ex-members of Tropa de Malaca, maintained the latter's core material but added new Portuguese dances learned from videotapes or cassettes and modified versions of two Fr. Sendim dances. Finally, Tropa de Assunta's comparatively limited repertoire consists almost entirely of material arranged by its leader, Stephen Theseira. By avoiding core repertoire and the more recently imported material, the Praya Lane group has emphasized both its separation from the Settlement "tradition" and its self-ascribed status as a *Malaysian*-Portuguese cultural troupe. Only one item—the *branyo*—is performed by all four groups. Omitted from the following tables because it predates the cultural dance repertoire and will be discussed separately below, the *branyo* is performed as a choreographed dance by Tropa de Malaca and Tropa de Assunta but as an audience-participation social dance by Rancho Folclorico San Pedro and (occasionally) by D'Tiru-Tiru.

Considering the foreign origin of the bulk of the repertoire (see table 1), it might seem odd that dances (tunes, texts, and choreography) introduced during the 1950s have been accepted as "ours," while the more recently imported material remains conceptually "Portuguese." This distinction sheds fascinating light on the changing construction of (and criteria for) authenticity within the developing tradition. Although core dances have gradually become part of the cultural heritage through which the Settlement-as-housing-estate derives its contemporary identity, they were, as we have already seen, introduced in the dying days of the colonial era by upper-class Eurasians seeking to distance themselves from the British and align themselves—not too closely—with a disadvantaged minority (the "poor Portuguese fisherfolk"). Instead of embracing the *branyo* tradition of their hybridized brethren, however, the Upper Tens chose to adopt dances they re-created from published sources as acceptable markers of non-British European identity. Despite the desire to reinvent themselves, upper-class Eurasians were still strongly British in their cultural orientation and placed great value on the authority vested in published sources. In fact, Christie Rodrigues insisted that these core dances were "authentic dances"—her choice of words—*because* they were learned from books (CRK, March 19, 1991). And a book like Armstrong's *Dances of Portugal* was particularly authoritative not only because it was British, but also because—as stated prominently on the title page—it was "published under the auspices of the Royal Academy of Dancing and the Ling Physical Education Association," an association that (in Bruner's 1994 terms) served to "duly certify" the authenticity of the book's contents.

As the Upper Tens faded from the social scene after independence, the dance group and its repertoire were taken over by Settlement residents. The transition from participants who were musically literate to those who were not precipitated significant changes in processes of acquisition and transmission, in turn affecting notions of authenticity and authority. First, new material was created locally rather than re-created from published sources (see table 2), and second, the entire repertoire (pre-existing core dances and newly composed material) began to be passed on orally to new performers. In consequence, authority was no longer vested in the written word (or note) but in a direct human link to Clement de Silva. Even today, surviving members of the first Settlement dance group consider their versions of core songs and dances to be "more authentic" than those of performers who did not learn directly from Clement de Silva.[3]

More recently imported material has not yet been incorporated into this authenticating human chain (see table 3). Although the dances were connected to the Upper Tens through Christie Rodrigues (Clement's sister-in-law), they were neither re-created from books nor locally composed. Instead, they were brought directly from Portugal by an eyewitness, Rodrigues herself. Each time she visited Portugal, she looked for interesting dances, recorded the music, and made a note of the choreography. Back in Malacca, she taught the dances to Fr. Sendim's group while Joe Lazaroo learned the music from her tapes. In a musicologist's eyes, this might confer more authority on the recently imported dances: they were, after all, learned in Portugal at first hand and not mediated by third parties (some of whom—like Armstrong—were not even Portuguese). In the eyes of Settlement residents, however, the direct link to Portugal is immaterial. Still associated with a single modern group, Rancho Folclorico San Pedro, the Sendim-Rodrigues dances remain foreign to the Settlement community because they have no local lineage. In effect, these dances have not yet become part of the canon.

The "our music"/"Portuguese music" distinction also draws our attention to the nature of the dances themselves. It is easy to assume that core and locally composed and choreographed dances are "folk dances": their straightforward musical accompaniments (using primarily I, IV, and V chords), simple steps, and uncomplicated formations give them the appearance of being rustic and thus "traditional."[4] In comparison, the Sendim-Rodrigues dances are musically and choreographically more virtuosic. Intended to be performed by trained musicians and dancers for tourist audiences in Portugal, these musically taxing and artistically choreographed show pieces emphasize fast tempos, a broader harmonic palette (including modulations), lifts, crisp turns, and sudden changes of direction. Of course, in Portugal the difference between folk and folkloric dances would have affected both the context in which particular dances were performed and the people who performed them. In Malacca, however, all the dances are performed on stage by cultural groups; none have been taken up by ordinary residents for their own celebrations. The difference between folk and folkloric dances in the Settlement was illustrated by Freddie Scully when he experimented with two Sendim-Rodrigues dances ("Minha Rosinha" and "Vira di Sta. Marta"). Instead of trying to compete with the speed and precision of Rancho Folclorico San Pedro, he slowed down their tempos, simplified their steps, and replaced their Portuguese texts with Kristang lyrics. The only other dances added to the repertoire (by Scully after 1985) also emphasize this seemingly "older" style of village folk dancing.[5]

Songs

As diverse and complex as the dance repertoire, songs can be divided into the same three subcategories: Portuguese songs learned during the 1950s by members of the Upper Tens from published sources; locally composed or arranged songs associated with the Portuguese Cultural Society period; and songs introduced since 1974. Despite the parallel process of accretion, songs from the 1950s have not remained part of the core repertoire of cultural groups.[6] Only two, "Os Marinheiros" and "Ala Marinheiros," are occasionally performed in public by Noel Felix and his musicians when strolling in hotel restaurants without the dance group. Locally composed songs have fared much the same: Noel Felix and Joe Lazaroo both perform their own songs when strolling but rarely use them in the context of cultural shows.[7] Only Tropa de Assunta, with its emphasis on Stephen Theseira's arrangements, uses local material on a regular basis.[8]

The songs selected from the available pool thus reflect more intimately the personal preferences of the two leading group leaders. Joe Lazaroo commands an enormous repertoire of sentimental Portuguese songs and *fados* learned over the years from Fr. Sendim and more recently from recordings and exchanges with Portuguese visitors. Noel Felix, less interested in Portuguese material (which he readily says he does not understand), has developed a more eclectic corpus, mixing 1950s Portuguese songs, his own compositions and cover versions, one recently imported Portuguese song ("Vinyo Verde"), and six songs learned from a cassette of popular songs from Macau.[9] Despite the wealth of material from which to draw, however, both singers consistently rely on a few favorites in the context of cultural shows.[10]

Footprints from the Past, Echoes from the Diaspora

Tracing the point at which various items entered the Settlement repertoire is only part of the story, of course. Each song or dance brings to the stage its own history, its own individual web of past associations that link the Settlement to the Portuguese diaspora across time and space. Even though musicians and dancers are rarely aware of these past lives, individual members of the audience may recognize particular associations. As Bruner (1994, 410) observed of Lincoln's New Salem (a reconstructed tourist site in Illinois), "Tourists are not monolithic, and neither is the meaning of the site." Although a complete inventory of all possible associations is clearly beyond the scope of this study, a limited sample can illustrate the variety of associations evoked and the range of diasporic connections activated. To this end, I have chosen three pieces—a song and two dances— as paradigmatic examples. Performed exclusively by Noel Felix, the song "Mama-să Filu" well illustrates the unexpected ways in which diasporic connections continue to ripple outwards. The dances "Jinkly Nona" and "Ti' Anika," in contrast, have both in different ways become "signature tunes" of the Settlement (see Sarkissian 1995–96). As we shall see, however, they are emblems that highlight the inherent ambiguity of its existence.

"Mama-să Filu"

Unlike much of the repertoire, we know exactly how and when "Mama-să Filu" reached the Settlement (see ex. 1, below on p. 164). It was introduced in 1986 by Noel Felix when he returned from the first Tropa de Malaca and Rancho Folclorico San Pedro tour to Macau. While in Macau, Noel bought a souvenir cassette, simply called *Macau,* of *tuna* (string band) music popular at the time on the island.[11] He was particularly attracted to the songs because the lyrics—attributed to the Macanese poet, José dos Santos Ferreira—were set in *papia Macau,* a kindred language easily understood by Kristang speakers. Noel quickly adopted two of the songs, "Asi-să Macau" and "Mama-să filu," as regular opening items in Tropa de Malaca cultural shows, invariably introducing both as songs from Macau. But while "Asi-să Macau" does celebrate famous sites around the tiny island, "Mama-să filu" is not a Macanese song at all; it turns out to be a local cover version of the well-known Brazilian song, "Mama Eu Quero."[12]

Closer inspection shows that in spite of its comparatively short history in Malacca, "Mama-să Filu" has one of the most convoluted pasts of the entire repertoire. The original version, "Mama Eu Quero," was recorded by Carmen Miranda during her first U.S. recording session (for Decca on December 26, 1939) and filmed the following year in her Hollywood debut, *Down Argentine Way* (Cardoso 1978, 473). The movie performance of this particular song introduced the world to the now-classic image of Carmen Miranda: the glamorous nightclub singer with bare midriff wearing a long flowing skirt, tight at the hips, and sporting a fruit-laden turban on her head. It also marked the beginning of the song's transformation. Performed by a Brazilian singer in a movie set in Argentina, "Mama Eu Quero" was no longer a purely Brazilian song; it became associated with South America in general. This impression was reinforced by subsequent comic versions of the song: Chico and Harpo Marx performed it as a piano duet in *The Big Store* (1941), while Mickey Rooney and Jerry Lewis both impersonated Carmen Miranda singing it in *Babes on Broadway* (1941) and *Scared Stiff* (1953), respectively.[13]

The song is also quickly recognized by baby boomers who grew up on a diet of American TV sitcoms.[14] In an early episode of *I Love Lucy* ("Be a Pal," which aired on October 22, 1951), Lucy was worried about her husband Ricky, who seemed to be depressed. On the advice of a pop psychology book provided by next-door-neighbor Ethel, Lucy decided to recreate Ricky's boyhood home in Cuba and to turn herself into (her vision of) his mother. When Ricky returned from work, he walked into a living room filled with what Lucy considered suitable reminders of his home: bunches of bananas, a stuffed donkey, and Ethel wearing a moustache, poncho, and large sombrero. Lucy entered—to Ricky's amazement—dressed as Carmen Miranda (right down to the costume and the fruit on her head) and lip synched to Miranda's recording of "Mama Eu Quero." This highly specific past association removes the song even further from its Brazilian roots. One of a series of stereotypical images in a white American middle-class vision of Cuba, "Mama Eu Quero" is transformed into an ambiguous marker of generic Latin identity. When Noel Felix steps onto a stage he is unaware of these (or other possible) past associations. And yet, each time he sings "Mama-să Filu," the ghosts of Carmen Miranda and Lucille Ball are revived, effectively linking Settlement residents and individual members of the audience together in multiple diasporic permutations.

"Ti' Anika"

"Ti' Anika's"[15] associations—while not as colorful as those of "Mama-să Filu"—are nevertheless remarkably diverse, linking the Settlement to the Portuguese diaspora temporally as well as geographically. Like most folk dances, "Ti' Anika's" origins are unknown, though textual references to place names (Loulé and Fuzeta) suggest that it comes from the southern part of the Algarve region.[16] Whatever its origins, inclusion in João do Rio's 1909 Brazilian publication *Fados, Songs, and Dances from Portugal* proves that "Ti' Anika" has been a world traveler for almost a century; it continues to connect modern Portuguese communities as far apart as Malaysia, Brazil, Hawai'i, and Perth, Australia.[17]

The exact details surrounding "Ti' Anika's" introduction to Malacca remain a mystery, although both Ida de Silva and Christie Rodrigues think it was learned from a book in the early days of the Upper Tens dance group (IRS, January 1, 1991; CRK, March 19, 1991). Since its first appearance on concert programs (ca. 1953), "Ti' Anika" has become a favorite core dance, one of the few performed by all Settlement groups. Indeed, it has become a sort of signature tune, surpassing even "Jinkly Nona," which, as we shall see below, has been rendered less ethnically distinctive because of its national associations. If there is time for only one dance to represent the community—say, in a TV soundbite or on a shared stage—it is usually "Ti' Anika." Despite its popularity, "Ti' Anika" remains firmly part of the cultural show: neither a social dance nor a village folk dance, this Settlement favorite is performed exclusively for the entertainment of outsiders.[18]

"Ti' Anika's" web is not limited solely to the Portuguese diaspora; it also forms a bridge between the Settlement and the broader Malaysian public. For many Malaysians, the cultural groups are the most prominent public feature of the Malaysian-Portuguese community and may be drawn upon in various ways to represent the community. For example, when—in an attempt to be politically correct and culturally inclusive—the choreographers of the state government-sponsored professional troupe Briged Seni Negeri Melaka (Malacca State Cultural Brigade)[19] developed a cultural show that juxtaposed dances from each of Malacca's ethnic minorities with regional Malay dances, they chose "Ti' Anika" as their token Malacca-Portuguese dance. Although Briged Seni's choreography is original, thus distancing this version from any particular Settlement version, the stereotypically Portuguese costumes and dance movements combined with the familiar tune (given additional jauntiness with mariachi-style trumpets) produce a version of "Ti' Anika" that is new yet instantly familiar. Although most Malaysians are unlikely to know the tune by name, "Ti' Anika" is easily recognized as an emblem of the Malaysian-Portuguese community (see ex. 2 on p. 165).

Now that cultural dance has become a prime means of promoting multicultural values in Malaysian schools, this particular bridge extends beyond professional troupes and into the classroom. For example, in a 1990 performance of "Ali Baba and His Forty Thieves" (endearingly entitled "Tin Pan Ali") given by students of a Kuala Lumpur grade school, the plot was interrupted by a short cultural show. After a Chinese lion dance performed by older children, a group of tiny children took to the stage in "Portuguese" costume. The choreography, most likely arranged by a school teacher, was simple, but the dance was "Ti' Anika" and the voice on the accompanying tape was clearly that of Joe Lazaroo.[20]

"Jinkly Nona"

"Jinkly Nona," the sole musical link between the prosaic everyday world of the Settlement-as-housing-estate and the magical onstage world of the Settlement-as-historical-monument, also marks the community's essential hybridity, knitting the Settlement into the Malaysian neighborhood as well as connecting it to the Portuguese diaspora. It is hardly surprising, then, that this *branyo* tune has the most complex history of my three examples. Its text has been found from one end of the Portuguese Asian diaspora to the other: as Edgar Knowlton reported in 1964, "Jingli Nona . . . a very popular song . . . was sung for me last February by a group of Malaccan children. A month later, Miss A. Margarida Gomes of Macau sang it to me in her home, and a week ago I learned that it is a popular song in Ceylon, where it is sung to Sinhalese words" (Knowlton 1964, 241). The connection exists across time as well as space: the first verse of the text from Malacca, as transcribed by Knowlton, is remarkably similar to a version recorded in Sri Lanka by C. M. Fernando (1894):

Malacca, 1964
(Knowlton 1964)

Malacca, 1991

Jingli nonă jingli nonă	Sinhalese girl, Sinhalese girl	*Jinkly Nona, Jinkly Nona*
Yo kerê kazá	I want to marry (you)	*Yo keré kazá*
Kază num tem portă	(Your) house has no door	*Kaza nunteng potra, Nona*
Ki laia logu pasá?	How (am I) to enter?	*Kái logu pasá?*

Sri Lanka
(Fernando 1894)

Cingalee Nona! Cingalee Nona!	Sinhalese girl, Sinhalese girl!
Eu kere kasa	I want to marry you
Porta ninkere, orta ninkere	I do not want your house or garden
Figa namas da	Just give (me) your daughter

The broad geographical distribution of the "Jinkly Nona" text, the lack of recent contact between locations in which it occurs, and the use in Malacca of rarely used Portuguese words in an otherwise Kristang text *(minya,* "my," is used in the chorus instead of the more common Kristang word, *yossa),* together suggest that this is an older song even if it does not date all the way back to Portuguese times.[21] And yet, as the title attests, the past to which it points is a mixed-race diasporic past, not a pure-blood Portuguese past. In the present-day Settlement, "Jinkly Nona" is glossed (if it is glossed at all) as "beautiful young girl with jingle bells on her ankles." But who is the girl? The ankle bells suggest that she is of Indian origin, an interpretation supported by Knowlton, David Jackson, and others, who gloss "Jinkly Nona" as "Sinhalese Girl." This is supported by Alan Baxter: when he worked with older Kristang speakers in 1980, *tera jingli* referred to "Ceylon" (Baxter pers. comm., July 12, 1999). Jackson also makes note of another version recounted in December 1987 by Francis Paynter, a creole speaker from Vypeen Island, Cochin, who was "of the opinion that 'Shingly' refers to the coastal city of Cranganur, citing K. L. Bernard's *Flashes of Kerala History.*" Paynter adds that the "name is said to mean 'little China,' because of the early Chinese trade and presence in Kerala" (Jackson 1990, 26):

Vypeen Island, Cochin
(Jackson 1998)

Shingly Nona, Shingly Nona	Chinese lady, Chinese lady
Eu kara casa	I want to marry you
Casa notha, Porta notha	I have no house, no door
Kalai lo casa	How shall we marry?

Whether of Indian, Sinhalese, or Chinese origin, it seems clear that the beautiful young subject of the song is an exotic local woman desired as a bride by her Portuguese suitor.

The complex web of diasporic and domestic connections is further illustrated in "Jinkly Nona's" formal structure, an open-ended series of four-line verses separated by a recurring chorus. In traditional practice, these verses, which were called *mata kantiga* (Kristang: "to kill the song"), were exchanged in a duelling fashion by male-female pairs of singers. After the standard opening "Jinkly Nona" verse, singers could either extemporize new material or draw upon an established body of stock quatrains, which could be used in conjunction with other *branyo* tunes. Each partner tried to outwit the other with verses that were romantic, flirtatious, scolding, or humorous in content. On the one hand, this structure, described by Isabel Tomás as *cantiga ao desafio* (where *desafio* means "challenge" and implies competition between male-female pairs of singers), links the Settlement to similar Portuguese duelling genres found as far afield as Brazil (Tomás pers. comm., November 15, 1990). On the other hand, the structural similarity between *mata kantiga* and *dondang sayang* (a Malay genre associated with the Malacca region and thought to be of Portuguese origin), provides firm evidence of long-standing domestic cross-fertilization. In fact, *mata kantiga* and *dondang sayang* are so much alike that older singers (e.g., Noel Felix and the late Rosil de Costa) were able to switch easily from one genre to the other simply by changing language.[22]

Unlike *dondang sayang*, which has its own distinctive melody and rhythmic pattern, *mata kantiga* verses are usually sung to the accompaniment of *branyo* dance tunes. This popular Settlement social dance is practically indistinguishable from the equally popular Malay social dance, *joget*. As Noel Felix says, "we say *branyo;* Malay, they say *joget*" (NF, July 5, 1991). Indeed, Malay *joget* tunes are frequently called *branyos* when performed at Settlement celebrations and, conversely, *branyo* tunes (like "Jinkly Nona") are called *jogets* when performed by Malay musicians. "Jinkly Nona" in particular has achieved a certain national celebrity, appearing frequently on cassette compilations of Malay *joget* tunes. In the process, however, it has lost its exclusivity: as Malacca's (now former) deputy state secretary, Cik Mohammed bin Saib, put it, "'Jinkly Nona' is more Malaysian than strictly Portuguese, because the Malays do it, the Portuguese do it, the Babas [Straits-born Chinese] do it, even the Indians do it" (MBS, April 3, 1991). Another Malay friend remembered singing it around camp fires as a boy without knowing of any Portuguese connection. The close connection between *joget* and Portuguese music is supported by scholars like Chopyak (1986, 124), who notes that the "joget dance form was greatly influenced by Portuguese and Malaysian Portuguese dancers and musicians from the time of the Portuguese occupation of Melaka, 400 years ago, until the present." That Portuguese influence on *joget* (and on *dondang sayang,* too, for that matter) is generally accepted but never precisely defined further reinforces their deep interconnectedness. This interaction has culminated both in the adoption of *joget* as the national social dance and the widespread acceptance of "Jinkly Nona" as national, rather than purely Settlement, property.

Musically, then, *branyo* in general and the tune "Jinkly Nona" in particular seem to cement the link between the Settlement and the broader Malaysian community. But again, this is not the whole story, for "Jinkly Nona" also provides a musical connection to the Portuguese Asian diaspora. The same tune, from Vypeen Island, Cochin, appears as Track 21 on the compact disc *Desta Barra Fora: Damão, Diu, Cochim, Korlai.* According to David Jackson's liner notes, the recording—made "more than thirty years ago, when many speakers of the Creole were still alive"—was discovered in 1993 by Francis Paynter (Jackson 1998, 57). In addition to knowing that the "Jinkly Nona" tune is sung elsewhere in the diaspora, there is also published evidence that it has existed for over a century: the first tune transcribed in C. M. Fernando's 1894 article on the traditional music of the Portuguese Mechanics of Ceylon is none other than "Singalee Nona" (see ex. 3 on p. 166).[23]

Processes of Domestication

Although the stage provides a forum for fleeting references to a Portuguese diaspora, these echoes are slowly being eclipsed as oral transmission and repeated performance gradually transform the repertoire (particularly the items classified as "our music") into something uniquely local. As texts and choreography of the diaspora are honed over time, it is becoming increasingly difficult to recognize the imported originals or even to distinguish between foreign and locally created material. In the process of domestication, new stories are created to bind the songs and dances to the Settlement; through repetition, they become part of the larger story residents tell about themselves and, ultimately, contribute in their own small way to the rewriting of history. While melodies continue to connect songs and dances to their diasporic pasts, there has, of course, been some musical domestication. Songs and dances are now played on whatever instruments are available—whether guitars, Malay *rebana* (frame drum), and mouth-organ or, more recently, electric guitars, synthesizers, and trap sets—by musicians who are equally adept at Malay *jogets,* country-western numbers, golden oldies, and the latest top-40 hits.

Stories

In its most common tourist-oriented form outside the Settlement, the cultural show comprises a medley of contrasting songs and dances. There may be a printed program or an emcee to give the spectators basic information—the title of a piece, where it comes from, and perhaps a detail or two for added color—but, for the most part, audience attention is directed away from potential language problems and toward a purely aural-visual smorgasbord. This type of cultural show, while generally common in Malaysia, is antithetical to Settlement practice.[24] Settlement cultural group leaders prefer to address the audience directly, introducing each item on the program in a manner in keeping with their own individual character. Sometimes their introductions tell a story that appears to contextualize and give color to the item about to be performed. Of course, the fact that Portuguese texts are not always fully understood by the performers leads to some interesting discrepancies between Settlement-created vignettes and the texts themselves. For example, Joe Lazaroo introduces the song "O Cochicho" with a vignette that describes young men sitting around, whistling at beautifully dressed young girls as they walk along the roadside (see chapter 5, time index 7.06 in the table). The Portuguese text actually tells a more dramatic story set amid the chaos and excitement of a festival parade: a narrator draws our attention to the sound of a whistle played by a girl and asks which of the lads wants to blow it. The girl, who has other ideas, relates fending off an unwanted suitor while stating firmly that her whistle will not be given to anyone (translated in Sarkissian 1998b, 104–105).

Other introductions appear to add a historical dimension but actually further domesticate the songs and dances by suggesting—sometimes obliquely—a long-term association with the Settlement. Freddie Scully, the leader who prided himself most on his skill as an emcee, was particularly adept at this kind of manipulation. Over the course of a show, Freddie adroitly seesawed between introductions that alluded to the age of a particular item and those that knitted the text into the fabric of Settlement lives. For example, early in a typical program, Freddie would inform the audience that "'O Vira Vamos' is a dance more than one or two centuries old, but it's still popular in Portugal." He states directly that the song is (in his opinion, at least) old, but cleverly sidesteps committing himself to the duration of its presence in the Settlement. A few dances later, he announces that "Ti' Anika" is "about a little old lady—'Little Aunty Annie'—a very short old lady, a popular figure in our community in the Good Old Days," this time locating the dance in a gently nostalgic past and firmly rooting it in the Settlement community. By the time he introduces "Fara Pera," the cumulative effect of his narrative detail has the audience convinced not only that this particular old dance had been a favorite *in the Settlement* for the past century, but also that he was recounting a piece of local folklore:

> It's a very, very old favorite. This is one of the very, very old dances, I should say more than a century, and it's called "Fara Pera." "Fara Pera" has got something to do with a beggar begging clothes for the poor community, but instead of being commented [*sic*] for his good work, he's been accused of begging these clothes for his personal self. But in the end, they found out that he was really doing a good job for his fellow beggars. As a result, we have this dance in his honor.

Texts

As is common in orally transmitted traditions, texts learned by ear and committed to memory are gradually transformed over time. This form of domestication is particularly common when, as is the case in the Portuguese Settlement, texts originally existed in an unfamiliar language. From the start, Clement de Silva taught the Settlement youngsters to memorize texts by rote, but as far as Josephine de Costa remembers, he never told them what the words meant (JTC, July 1, 1991).[25] Unable to make complete sense of the Portuguese lyrics, singers generally employ one of two strategies: approximation or substitution. These strategies can be seen by comparing the following two versions of "Ti' Anika."[26] The first version, a typescript from the collection of Joe Lazaroo, records the text as it was taught to Settlement residents by Clement de Silva in the early 1950s. With a written text to refresh his memory, Joe's version remains closer to the "original." The second version—my transcription of Noel Felix's rendition of the song—only exists orally. The English translation is based on Joe's written text; it is impossible to translate Noel's version of the text.

Joe Lazaroo		*Noel Felix*
(typed, n.d.)		(oral, 1990)

Olé, olá	*Olé, olá*	*Olé, olá*
Esta vida não está má	This life's not so bad	*Engsabida nus toma*
Olá, olé	*Olá, olé*	*Olá, olé*
Ti Anica de Loulae	Aunty Annie from Loulé	*Ti' Anika di lolay*
Ti' Anica, Anica	Aunty Annie, Annie	*Ti' Anika, Anika*
Ti' Anica de Fuzeta	Aunty Annie from Fuseta	*Ti' Anika ja fuzayta*
A quem desejaria ela	I wonder to whom she gave	*Agienda ira ela*
Asaia da bara preta	The skirt with the black border	*Azianda bara preta*
Olé, olá, etc.	*Olé, olá, etc.*	*Olé, olá, etc.*
Asaia da bara preta	The skirt with the black border	*Azianda bara preta*
A bara do cachine	The edging of ?	*Abaranda kashiné*
Ti' Anica, mana'nica	Aunty Annie, sister Annie	*Ti' Anika manda'nika*
Ti' Anica de Loulae	Aunty Annie from Loulé	*Ti Anika di lolay*
Olé, olá, etc.	*Olé, olá, etc.*	*Olé, olá, etc.*

As the example shows, it is not only "esoteric ritual speech . . . that is 'broadcast but not understood' by the general populace" (Aragon 1996, 422). Noel Felix's most frequently employed strategy for dealing with unfamiliar words is to approximate their sounds—e.g., "agienda ira" for "a quem desejaria," "engsabida" for "esta vida," and "azianda" for "asaia da." This results in the creation of new vocabulary, most of which has no meaning in either Portuguese or Kristang. Occasionally, when the original text has been forgotten, Noel substitutes familiar Kristang words or phrases, whether or not they bear any relation to the content of the surrounding lyrics—e.g., "nus toma" ("we take") for "não está má," or "ja" ("already," a tense-aspect participle) for "de." Noel's explanation of his text creatively takes the process of domestication one step further and leads to a completely new storyline:

> Auntie Annie, I ask you where have you been? *Agienda* is something to do with the tide, a flood. *Agienda ira ela, azianda bara preta*—there's a flood on the east side. *Engsabida nus toma* means "whose name we take." *Kashiné*

is "don't bother at all." *Azianda bara preta, abaranda kashineh*—even
though there's a flood on the east side, we don't have to bother anything.
(NF, November 14, 1990)[27]

Textual domestication began as a practical response to the unfamiliar
vocabulary of an imported repertoire. Over the years, however, it has become an organic part of the now-local tradition. Although Kristang-
dominant singers (e.g., Noel Felix) began the process of "smoothing
out" the words, other singers—ranging from Kristang-dominant singers
who trace their texts directly to Clement de Silva (e.g., Josephine de Costa)
to English-dominant singers who tend to stick more closely to the written
word (e.g., Joe Lazaroo)—have also introduced their own personal idio-
syncrasies. Today, each singer has his or her own unique version of core-
repertoire Portuguese texts. These texts continue to diverge as second-
and third-generation singers pick them up orally. In the case of "Fara
Pera" (ex. 4, on p. 167), for example, Joe Lazaroo's text remains
relatively faithful to the Portuguese original (as published in Leça ca.
1983).[28] The version performed by Josephine's son Gerard de Costa, in
contrast, has been so thoroughly domesticated that the original text is
barely recognizable and the resultant text cannot be translated. Like
his mentor, Noel Felix, Gerard frequently substitutes Kristang phrases
(e.g., *nus tă kantá tă balá,* "we are singing and dancing") that have nothing to do with the subject of the original text. Not even Gerard himself
could identify the words he used in the line and a half of text marked
"unclear."

Leça
(published, ca. 1983)

Chamaste-me farrapeira	Call me *farrapeira*
Eu nunca vendi farrapos	I never sold old clothes
Tenho uma camisa nova	I have a new shirt
Toda cheia de buracos	That's all full of holes

Joe Lazaroo	*Gerard de Costa*
(oral, 1990)	(oral, 1991)
[chorus]	[chorus]
A e o lay (× 4)	*A e o lay (× 4)*

Chamastema fara pera

Yo nungka vendi perapus

A e o lay

Yo nungka vendi perapus

Teng ungwa saia nova

Toda chea di burakos

Chamastema fara pera

Yo nungka vendi perapus

[chorus]

A e o lay (× 4)

O minya fara peresta

O minya fara perona

A e o lay

Fara pera

[unclear]

[unclear] alegra

O minya pera

Nus tă kantá tă balá

[chorus]

A e o lay (× 4)

Choreography

It is much harder to judge the extent to which choreography has been domesticated. While it might be possible to compare current versions of particular dances with the versions introduced by the Upper Tens in the 1950s or by Christie Rodrigues in the 1970s (though fading memories and the firm conviction that one's own version is "authentic" tend to make this difficult), it is impossible to judge how closely any of these dances resemble Portuguese originals as they existed at the moment of introduction. All the core dances introduced by the Upper Tens were mediated in some way, most commonly by folk dance collectors who published their own interpretations of particular dances; the second wave of Portuguese dances, collected at first hand by Christie Rodrigues, were often reset by Rodrigues herself. Once again, in Settlement eyes "authenticity" is a quality traced, not back to Portugal, but to authoritative versions taught by Clement de Silva. Although there is clearly a fund of shared movements, the fact that all three Settlement groups perform distinct versions of core dances suggests that some domestication of choreography has occurred over time.

The possibility of choreographic domestication is greatly facilitated by the rapid turnover of dancers. While a small corps of dedicated dancers perform for several years, the performing life expectancy of most dancers is relatively short. All sorts of factors, including age, physical condition, school and/or job commitments, relationships, marriage, etc., ensure that dancers change frequently, spawning many more "generations" of dancers than of musicians or leaders. Since dances are passed from one dancer's body to the next, there is plenty of scope for gradual transformation, although—like watching a flower grow—change is almost imperceptible. Occasionally, however, a situation arises in which change becomes visible. One such incident occurred at a Rancho Folclorico San Pedro rehearsal in June 1994. An old dancer who had trained under Christie Rodrigues returned to the Settlement and wanted to rejoin the group. He was invited to the practice, but his dancing no longer "fit": his turns were too fast, his hands were held too high above his head, his wrists were too tense, and his changes of direction were too sharp. The other dancers made smooth turns, the boys held their arms at ear height, their wrists were held in a limp, relaxed fashion, and their changes of direction involved a gradual slowing down before the actual turn. Circular running movements caused the most chaos: each time the other dancers slowed down before changing from clockwise to counterclockwise motion, the old dancer—who turned on a dime—crashed straight into the girl following him. The juxtaposition of an old dancer with a more recent group clearly showed that changes had occurred, despite the fact that the intervening generations of dancers thought they were transmitting the movements exactly as they had learned them. These changes are evidence not only of domestication but also of hybridization. One of the girls described the old dancer's movements with a Malay word: they were too *kasar,* too "rough." Without realizing it, Settlement dancers have gradually introduced the more *alus* ("refined") movements characteristic of Malay dance. In keeping with their mixed heritage, Portuguese dances performed by Settlement dancers have over time become "smooth" and infinitesimally more gracefully Malay.[29]

In addition to the gradual hybridization of dance movements, a broader sense of choreographic freedom is developing as younger-generation musicians and dancers are beginning to step into leadership roles. This embryonic tendency, so far only apparent within Tropa de Malaca (because Noel Felix has ceded day-to-day running of the group to Gerard de Costa), is reducing the emphasis placed on "authenticity" and the direct link to Clement de Silva. For young musicians and dancers, many of whose parents danced in their day, the cultural groups have always been part of Settlement life. For them, it is not so important to repeat exactly what they learned; doing that year after year is not only boring but also suppresses their own creativity. It is thus just as natural for them to experiment with cultural dance group choreography as it is for Settlement teens and pre-teens to create new synchronized moves for the latest dance craze. With an internalized vocabulary of basic Portuguese (or Portuguese-like) movements, Gerard de Costa and other members of Tropa de Malaca have begun working out what they call "new variations."

Erasing the Past

The increasing domestication of the once-imported tradition is, in many ways, an exciting development—a development reflective of the political realities of contemporary Settlement life. As imported and local elements are juxtaposed on stage, past associations are conjured up and eclipsed, and conflicting worlds converge and are fused. In the resulting synthesis, the songs and dances of the Settlement-as-historical-monument are becoming an organic expression of cultural life in the Settlement-as-housing-estate. At the same time, however, this bridge to the imagined world of D'Albuquerque is erasing a more recent past, a hybrid past that links the Settlement to its Malaysian neighbors. This particular past is musically rooted in the *branyo*. Although it is still the favorite social dance of the Settlement, the *branyo* has changed considerably over the period during which the cultural dance tradition has developed. Younger-generation musicians view these changes as modernization or the creative adaptation of a living tradition to new social contexts. *Branyo*s are still played at Settlement celebrations, only now they are sandwiched between the latest hits and played by pop bands using electric guitars, keyboards, and trap set (replacing the old-fashioned hybrid ensemble of violin and Malay *rebana*). And *branyo*s still connect the Settlement to its neighbors, only now young musicians bolster their limited repertoire with popular Malay *joget*s, which they sing either with new Kristang lyrics (e.g., "Joget Selayang Pandang," known in the Settlement as "Langgiang, Langgiang"), or in Malay (e.g., "Joget Pahang"), or even in a humorous mixture of English and pidgin Tamil (e.g., the Chitty Melaka *joget*, "Jingali Jingalay"). In contrast, older residents, who remember the excitement of the song duel, the plethora of *mata kantiga* quatrains, and the many subtypes of *branyo*, view the same changes as evidence of the impoverishment of a once vital tradition.

In its heyday, *branyo* was the primary entertainment of the Settlement. No celebration or festival was complete without singing and dancing, and everyone was expected to extemporize a *mata kantiga* verse or two. Often the verses were flirtatious or humorous, but sometimes—when the rice alcohol began to take effect—they became a way for neighbors to air grievances in a socially sanctioned forum. Considered low-brow by polite society, the only contemporaneous references to *branyo* parties that reached the newspapers focused on the occasional public disturbances. Omission from the historical record has, of course, speeded up the process of erasure, and, as older residents pass away, the pool of oral testimonies is steadily diminishing. The following eyewitness account, related by Noel Felix (b. 1930), vividly captures the flavor of Settlement social life and the passing of the old-time *branyo:*

NF: When I was young day, ah, there is a festival and, you know, they will have this kind of *branyo* and so on and whatnot. But we are not supposed to join, because we are young. You see, if we go in and disturb the thing, we might get slapped from the old peoples and we might be chased out.

MS: What kind of festival? Like San Pedro, or what?

NF: San Pedro, ah yes, they have the *branyo* all. Christmas, all sometimes they have, after Christmas they have the *branyo* celebration. The San Pedro is grand. They only have, like, this carnival in the sea, you know. They have this boat racing, they have the sailing boat and so forth. And then they'll have a BIG boat, no [you know], this *tongkan nadé* they call. All the old folks, no, and say, above 30-*lah* the people, the women and men. They above 30, because most of them are married that time. So they'll go into the *nadé* from Pulau Jawa [a nearby island]—from here they'll go to Pulau Jawa—and from Pulau Jawa, they'll come, they'll play the *branyo* inside the *nadé.* They will be dancing all! And you can see the liquor all in their pouch, no. They use *sarong kebaya,* those days, they have. So they, the ladies drinking like a man!

MS: Is it?

NF: Yes! But the liquor is not like nowadays. The liquor all they make on their own one. The *pulut* [Malay: "rice"], they make they liquor. But they really get drunks and they enjoy. So they come to the land and they start dancing until midnight! And then boat will be blessing in the evening. After that, the best decoration will get holy pictures. Big, small, first, second, third, and others will get consolation, the small holy pictures. That's all they get. But it was very grand, they celebrate.

MS: How old were you when they were celebrating like that?

NF: I was only about nine to ten years old. Very young. I used to watch. That's why I told you, we are not supposed to go in. We can only listening—they sing so nice, no, they sing! And they have got so many people who can *pantun* [Malay: extemporize verses],[30] and when they *pantun,* after few days, they have a fight! Because why-*lah,* it's something like hinting, no, so badly hinting, no. They fought. They fight. Because of the words, which is like—you know, sometimes they just simply bang you and then the fella cannot repeat back. So they kept for grudge-*lah*. After few days, they will fight, they quarrel. Is a very poison, no, these words. They say all kinds of things. Is about your personal feeling-*lah*. They will fire you. In the *branyo* itself they fire. Suppose they don't fight, they cannot fight the neighbor—when we went to the party, there's the time-*lah*. You will see me, I sing so, the singer all banging only!

ms: So you don't fight from day to day, you wait. . . .

nf: Ah, they wait until the celebration comes, so they bang each another. Is quite interesting, yes! So those days there were lot of violinists and singers. And all elderly people. But I'm so inquisitive, I'm so interested, no! So I still put in my nose a bit far away from them, by listening them what they are doing. So that's how I managed to, you know, do things by myself and follow the old people. Otherwise this thing is already dead, long time ago. . . . And then later, when I was eighteen years old, that's the time, the thing still on, but not, not that great as before-*lah*, what I mean. When I was growing up that time the thing is becoming slack.

ms: When you were listening, how old were you then?

nf: I was about nine. Nine, ten, eleven, twelve. Why I'm not supposed to join the party.

ms: You stand outside and listen.

nf: Yes. And then, when I became eighteen, nineteen, twenty, the thing, ah, getting slack, slack, slack, slack! All the violinists are dying. So there's no violin. All the people who can debate the song—all gone. Left Aunty Rosil. Aunty Rosil and myself was being very popular for some time. After Aunty Rosil died, left I alone. Nobody there. That's why my *pantun* is quite a lot. These people [younger-generation singers]—I love, I love to see they do things, because is good. Is something like replacement, you got me? But it's a pity they don't have much *pantun*. If they come with me and ask, I don't mind to give them, because they are young.

(NF, *July 18, 1996*)

In an earlier interview, Noel compared the depth of community involvement in the old-time *branyo* to the present situation, in which he sings alone. In the old days, residents were more familiar with the art of duelling. In fact, so many couples participated in the singing, that one could dance for an hour before having to sing again:

NF: I tell you, ah, when my youngest days—beautiful-*lah*! You see, when there's *branyo*, look at the *pantun*—from that end to this end! All know how to *pantun*. One fella sing one [verse]—is good enough already. You don't have to sing three or five. Like myself, I'm singing about 20 verses. No point! Just one will do. We have at least about 30, 40 fellas at the wedding, no, *mata kantigu* and *branyo*. You sing one, you can wait for one hour, the other fellas going continually. See, like—we dancing, before we dancing pairs, ah. Come to my turn, the girl will *pantun* and after the girl, I *balas* [Malay: "respond"] back. And then I forget about it, no, the thing going on only. And from that end, it come back to this end [he laughs]. The most we will sing about three or four verses only. But like now—where, where got people?

(NF, *June 30, 1991*)

Although a quick wit was highly valued, singers were not obliged to make up verses spontaneously. Most of the time, they drew upon an orally transmitted body of quatrains. In the late 1930s (roughly the same time Noel is describing above) Fr. António Silva Rêgo collected over 160 quatrains, which he classified by content and opening formula into three categories: *cantigas de amigo, cantigas de mal-dizer,* and *cantigas indiferentes.* According to Silva Rêgo (1941, 24–70), romantic *cantigas de amigo* often began with the formulaic line "Nona, minya Nona" ("Lady, my Lady") or "Passa Nona sa porta" ("Passing your door"), while insulting *cantigas de mal-dizer* began with "Ala banda esti banda" ("That place, this place"); his miscellaneous category, *cantigas indiferentes,* comprised nonformulaic quatrains that were neither romantic nor insulting. Although Silva Rêgo never acknowledged his sources, Alan Baxter has confirmed that two of his main informants were Rosil de Costa and her husband, Peter (pers. comm., July 12, 1999).

In the old days, experienced song duellers generally began with stock verses arranged with regard to textual continuity, but as they warmed up and started to react to each other's comments, responses became more original. In the following sequence, transcribed from Alan Baxter's 1980 recording of Rosil de Costa and Stephen Theseira, we can see this process clearly. Verses are split into two couplets, each of which is repeated (i.e., AABB); the chorus is sung after each verse by all present. Verses marked with an asterisk appear in Silva Rêgo's 1941 collection. The asterisk in parentheses (*) indicates a variant of a verse collected by Silva Rêgo. Towards the end, stock phrases initiate insults but improvised humor soon takes over again.

Chorus (all together):

Teng kántu teng	You've got what you've got
Kántu teng falá nunteng	However much you have, you say you have nothing
Amor minya amor	Amor, my love
Amor minya korsang	My love, my dear [lit.: "my heart"]

* Stephen:

Jinkly Nona, Jinkly Nona	Jinkly Nona, Jinkly Nona
Yo keré kazá	I want to marry you
Kaza nunteng potra[31] *Nona*	Your house has no door
Kái logu pasá?	How can I enter?

* Rosil:

Da lisensia Siára meu	Give me your permission
Yo rintá bos să jarding	That I may enter your garden
Rafinadu súa cheru	Your perfumed smell
Chuma roza menggaring[32]	Is like a jasmine flower

* Stephen:

O Nona minya Nona	Nona, my Nona
Ai Nona minya korsang	Nona, my dear
Ai Nona mutu bemfeta	You are very beautiful
Baba ja kai n(a)' afesang	I've fallen for your beauty

* Rosil:

Afesang nă afesang	The beauty of your beauty
Afesang grandi poderu	Beauty has such power
Yo pasá risku di motri	I will risk death
Sigi Nona să keré	To follow your desire[33]

Stephen:

Pai mai ńgka kontenti	Parents don't agree
Ki fazé keré kazá?	Why do we want to get married?
Tristi di bida	A sad life
Ai nos dos logu pasá	We'll both have

Rosil:

Baba ja sta kontenti	If you agree
Nona taming-lah kontenti	Then I'm also happy
Paski Nona lo bai lonzi	Even if I go far away
Nada kazá otru jenti	I won't marry anyone else

Stephen:

O Baba minya Baba	Baba, my Baba
Yo tă bai Alor Gajah[34]	I'm going to Alor Gajah
Kántu Nona ńgka konfiansá	If you don't believe me
Yo birá logu kazá	I'll come back and marry you

Rosil interrupts the chorus to comment "Sertu!" ("Sure you will!")

* Rosil:

Baba minya Baba	Baba, my Baba
Kái lonzi-lah bolu bai	However far you go
Si yo ńgka achá ku bos	If I don't get you
Nunka fila de 'nya mai	I'm not my mother's daughter

Stephen:

Pena tinta ja skribé	The ink pen has written
Ai súa letra bong bong finu	With fine handwriting
Si yo ńgka achá ku Nona	If I don't get you
Ki úngua grandi di mufinu	It'll be a great misfortune

* Rosil:

Pescador mia pescador	Fisherman, my fisherman
Pescador mutu fedé	You're very smelly
Pena tinta teng nă mang-lah	If there's a pen in your hand
Baba ku Nona lo keré	Then I want you

(*) Stephen:

O Baba minya Baba	Baba, my Baba
Ai sepatu gritá gritá	[I'm wearing] tap-dancing shoes
Pataka nteng nă saku	There's no money in my pocket
Dodo Nona kubisá[35]	Only a crazy woman would admire me

Rosil:

This entire verse is unclear. Rosil missed her cue, so the violinist covered as if taking a solo. Rosil entered one line later, but her words cannot be made out.

* Stephen:

Pasá Baba să potra	As I was passing your door
Tă ubi matá galinya	I heard a chicken being killed
Súa sanggi fazé tinta	It's blood makes ink
Súa letra ku raīnya	Your handwriting is like a queen's

The following is usually a man's verse; it doesn't completely make sense when Rosil sings it.

* Rosil:

Pasá Nona să potra	As I was passing you door
Pidi agu ke(ré) bebé	I asked for some water to drink
Raskundé Nona di drentu	You replied from inside
O mansebu, ki bos keré?	Young man, what do you want?

Stephen:

O Nona minya Nona	Nona, my Nona
Ai Nona minya korsang	Nona, my dear
Bela Bela mizá forsa	If you [old woman] pee forcefully
Fazé buraku nă chang	You'll make a hole in the ground

At this point the audience starts to laugh and urge Rosil to counter this insult. Unfortunately, the background encouragement becomes so loud that it is impossible to hear Rosil's response. It must have been good, judging from the laughter and admiring comments that follow.

* Rosil and Stephen:

Jinkly Nona, Jinkly Nona	Jinkly Nona, Jinkly Nona
Yo keré kazá	I want to marry you
Kaza nunteng potra Nona	Your house has no door
Kái logu pasá?	How can I enter?

As Noel Felix's account suggests, the old-fashioned *branyo* was already in decline by the time the cultural dance groups appeared in the early 1950s. The duelling style died out altogether after Rosil de Costa, the last female *branyo* singer, passed away in the early 1980s. Instead of engaging in flirtatious duels with young women, the best young male singers—like Josephine de Costa's son, Gerard—make an effort to collect and memorize fixed verses which they juxtapose without particular attention to textual continuity. Other singers randomly string a small number of memorized verses in between extemporized crude quatrains.[36] Alan Baxter has suggested that this might be another dimension of shrinkage and loss, noting that Aunty Rosil complained to him in 1980 about the increasing tendency to use crude texts (Baxter pers. comm., July 12, 1999).

In addition to the demise of the duelling style and the diminishing body of *mata kantiga* verses, older musicians also lament the disappearing musical tradition. Musical accompaniments have dwindled to the extent that the modern *branyo* is generally represented by a single melody, "Jinkly Nona."[37] In the past, it seems, there were many subtypes of *branyo,* including *sarampa, chikoti* (or *chikotri*), *bintana,* and *morisko.* Today these genres are almost moribund. Their names are still recognized, but only a few of the oldest musicians remember their tunes. There is very little consensus either on what the terms meant or on which tune was an example of which particular subtype. In his Kristang-English dictionary (1987), Baxter offers the following definitions: *bintana,* a type of *branyo; chikoti,* form of *mata kantiga; sarampa,* a *branyo* song type. Of all these terms only one—*chikoti*—is mentioned outside Malacca. Fernando briefly mentions *chikothi* in his account of the music of the Portuguese Mechanics of Sri Lanka. Contrasting it to the lively *cafferina,* he observes that "the slow measures of the 'Chikothi' only call for stately and dignified steps" (Fernando 1894, 187).

The existence of the subgenre called *morisko* remains a mystery. The term does not appear in Baxter's dictionary, but in the middle of a long discussion about old-style *branyos,* Noel Felix remembered two tunes he identified as fast and slow *moriskos.* At first, the absence of Kristang references to the term "morisko" seemed striking in light of Kornhauser's discussion of Moriscos (converted Moors absorbed into the Portuguese Christian community and who lived in a similar enclave called Tugu in Jakarta) and their influence on the development of Indonesian *kroncong* music. Neither of Noel's *moriskos* sounded like the tune Kornhauser (1978, 179–83) identified as "Kroncong Moritsku." Since the only person in the Portuguese Settlement who used the term was Noel Felix, Alan

Baxter has suggested it might have been introduced by way of an old correspondence between Noel and Jacobus Quiko, a Eurasian from Tugu (pers. comm., July 12, 1999).

The waters are further muddied by what appear to be subdivisions of the subtypes (e.g., *sarampa di monya, chikoti marindu,* and *chikoti mimuria*) or by tunes known by proper names (e.g., *sarampa* "Abri boka, rosa fala"; *branyo* "Tra lai ngoleng ngoleng"; "Kanji papa"). However, there is no longer any consistency to the terminology: Noel Felix categorizes *branyo* "Tra lai ngoleng ngoleng" (the first words of the chorus) as a *sarampa* and "Kanji papa" as a slow *bintana.* Another melody identified as a fast *bintana* by Noel Felix was called a *sarampa* by Georgie de Costa (of D'Tiru-Tiru) and *branyo di instrumintu* ("instrumental *branyo*") on a field recording by Baxter.[38] Some of this confusion is apparent in the following excerpt from a discussion with Noel Felix on the subject of the *branyo.* Despite his assertion towards the end of the conversation that *bintana* was slow and *sarampa* fast, Noel later contradicted himself by singing two *bintana*s (fast and slow), two *sarampa*s (fast and slow), and two *morisko*s (fast and slow).

nf: They make the name, these old people-*lah.* I don't know. We follow by the oldest people, you see. Even I don't make this song. They make. So we only follow only. They call this *sarampa,* this *bintana.*

ms: So "Jinkly Nona's" not *sarampa,* not *bintana*? Separate, eh?

nf: Separate. Because "Jinkly Nona" was the first *branyo* music, was originated by the Portuguese. That was the first. And then came the *bintana, sarampa di monya, chikotri,* all and so forth.

ms: *Sarampa di monya* is which one? The fast one or the slow one?

nf: *Sarampa di monya* is—what you call—the fast one just now. No—*sarampa di monya* is a bit slow. . . .

nf: You see, it's only if you put every time you play "Jinkly Nona," every time you play *sarampa,* people fed up. So they just say "*agora nossa bringka bintana*" [Kristang: "now we'll play *bintana*"]. After that they say "OK, *nos ta bringka, ki fala, sarampa*" ["OK, now we are playing— what's it called—*sarampa*"], then also "*bringka morisko*" ["play *morisko*"]. Just like that-*lah.* So, the name only different and the beat different. Because got slow, got fast—like that-*lah.* Like old lady normally they sing this *bintana,* why you know? *Bintana* is a very slow one. They can, because they got no stamina. Like we all young-young fellas, we sing *sarampa,* because *sarampa* is a fast one. *Sarampa* and "Jinkly Nona." [Sings] "O nona minya nona/Nona minya korsang" That is *sarampa,* fast one. . . .

NF: The branyo, if you want to know the meaning why this, this like that, is just like that-*lah.* Same like English songs—some people they like rock, some people they like waltz, some people they like rumba, something like that-*lah.* That's why they have the different-different beats.

(NF, *July 5, 1991*)

Of all the *branyo* subtypes, only a single fast *sarampa* melody can still be heard regularly—not spontaneously performed at community dances, but preserved in Tropa de Malaca cultural shows. Until our conversations on the subject, Noel Felix had not sung many of the old *branyo* subtypes in years; others, like the *chikoti,* he had completely forgotten. Although he defined genres by their characteristic rhythms, in practice there was no consistency to his examples. Whatever the truth of the matter, it is clear that this particular, somewhat confused, remnant of Settlement history will be completely erased when Noel Felix and the last few carriers pass away.

March 1991 With about an hour before Tropa de Malaca's evening performance, Noel's niece Maria and I are lazing around the air-conditioned hotel room watching the in-house video channel. It is the third time we've tried to watch the same Nick Nolte movie; each time we catch a different part. There's a knock on the door, and, as I open it, the phone rings. Anne, at the other end of the line, wants a decision on the evening's costume. Maria's older sister, Merina, and cousin Anita, just back from the afternoon poker session in their uncle's room, suggest the red and black set they call "full Macau." They used the velvet set at lunchtime and "half Macau" yesterday. Once agreed, everyone starts to change. The phone rings again: black or white stockings? Anita holds up her white pair to display a run in one leg. That settles it: black.

Everyone crowds around the mirror to check costumes and put on makeup. First one to finish helps the others. Talk is casual. No one mentions the performance. There is nothing much to be said. It's our third "Malacca Week" hotel food promotion in the last two months: Singapore, Penang, and now a beach resort on the east coast, outside the town of Kuantan. A busier than average season. It has been a relief to escape the chronic water shortage in Malacca, if only temporarily, but the novelty of hotel food, two shows a day, and endless gambling in between is wearing thin. There's not much else to do here. No friends to visit. No shops. No foodstalls open all hours. Nothing but the beach, and only *Ropiano dodo*—crazy Europeans—sit out in the hot sun. Anne, her younger sister Laura, and Anne's cousin-in-law Ubelda walk in from next door. 'Belda hasn't changed because it's her turn to babysit Carrieanne while Anne dances. Hats or headscarves? Hats look better with "full Macau" it's agreed, and anyway, the guys borrowed the headscarves earlier. It seems they want to try a "pirate" look tonight.

When everyone is ready we head for Uncle Noel's room. From the hall you can hear the commotion of last-minute preparations. The musicians appear first, and Gerard de Costa, Anne's husband, hands a guitar to his sister-in-law, Laura. Finally the dancers emerge, still straightening jackets and headscarves. They don't look much like pirates, but it's something different. Riding together in a single elevator, it's quite a crush—especially with three guitarists simultaneously trying to tune to my accordion. The sudden laughter is at Fabian's expense. Last night, clowning about on the way to the outdoor stage, he didn't notice an open drain and fell right in. Luckily no harm was done—a twisted ankle would have meant dancing with three couples instead of four. As we reach the lobby, Christopher mimes 'Bian's fall and the look of surprise on his face. It's exactly 8:30: showtime. After a brief pause to make sure everyone is ready, Noel leads the musicians in single file through the restaurant. The dancers, still laughing, follow in pairs holding hands.

As soon as we have finished adjusting the microphones, Noel starts the performance with two of his favorite songs, "Asi-să Macau" and "Mama-să filu." The dancers stand off to one side, but Merina's husband Gerard Lazaroo's enthusiastic hand-clapping, foot-stomping encouragement is infectious. The energy level is high tonight, despite the unusually small crowd in the restaurant. After the second song, the dancers move center stage, form a circle, and start swaying gently to the introduction of "Ti' Anika." As they start to move, gracefully weaving in and out of the circle, it becomes clear that Noel's pace is too slow for the boisterous mood. One of the dancers catches the eye of Benjamin, the drummer. Almost imperceptible nods and winks pass between 'Amin and the guitarists; the tempo increases, sweeping Noel and the rest of us along. As the applause subsides, everyone has to remain alert, for Noel is never truly predictable. While he usually sticks to familiar material (though he often varies the order), there is always the chance that he might start an old song that Laura and I haven't played before, necessitating quick sideways glances at the other guitarists' fingers (and lending a whole new meaning to the term "sight reading"). Or he might introduce one dance but begin to sing another, resulting in rapid redeployment on the dance floor.

Like any other momentary lapse, however, such slips are skillfully covered.

Occasionally someone's attention wanders: tonight Edward, the guitarist to my right, has noticed a *Ropiano* in the audience eyeing Laura. During one of the slower numbers he passes a wicked comment in mixed Malay and Kristang, just loud enough for all of us on stage to hear. Laura looks up shyly, blushes, and giggles. Edward's risqué remark is tossed around the floor until it becomes the catch phrase for the evening, a spontaneous shout of encouragement between musicians and dancers, and even Noel can't suppress the twinkle in his eye. Tonight everyone is in a good mood. After 45 minutes exactly, Noel wraps up with a choreographed *branyo* and calls it a night.

Back in the elevator, everyone—including Noel—teases Laura mercilessly. As 'Pher, the clown, impersonates her latest admirer, even shy, silent Jimmy laughs as we walk back to our rooms. Once inside, there's a flurry of activity as costumes are hung up to air and everyone starts to change. Conversation quickly turns to dinner and plans for the rest of the evening. It's Saturday night and there's a live band playing in the lounge. Laura has been asked to fill in because the regular Filipina singer is in Singapore renewing her visa. Edward will probably sing, too, and maybe— if we ply him with some beer first—'Amin will sing a few verses of "Jinkly Nona." Later, the dancers want to check out the hotel disco; the manager said he would overlook the cover charge as a treat. Anonymous out of their costumes and dancing to a different beat—M.C. Hammer is the current favorite—they know heads will still turn the moment they hit the dance floor.

● ● ●

Seemingly transparent, the cultural show is—like any theatrical performance—a fluid and complex construction in which the lines between reality and the imagined quickly become blurred. What is perceived as real and what is born of the imagination depend on who is doing the looking and why. Spectators in front of the stage see "the show," a bounded entity that they accept as more or less "authentic" depending on their individual expectations (see MacCannell 1973, 1992). From their perspective, the musicians and dancers become visible when they step onto the stage in costume and dance to Portuguese music. The opening vignette shows, however, that the view from the performer's perspective is quite different. As in the theatrical world in general, performers do not exist solely in the fleeting gaze of the audience. While performing is certainly a job—the musicians and dancers are professionals who coordinate their efforts in order to create a product that is sold (often indirectly) to outsiders—it is also part of everyday life: preparations are made beforehand, life continues afterwards, and even in the midst of the action, there is always time to interact outside the frame of the performance. Performing unites a circle of friends who express themselves artistically, state their identity as Malaysians of Portuguese descent in a socially and—more important—politically sanctioned arena, and most important of all, have fun together on as well as off stage.

The cultural show is a crucial part of what Bruner has called the "touristic borderzone" (1996), a special forum in which culture is invented and contested at multiple levels. In this "borderzone," as Boon has pointed out of Bali (the regional tourist sight/site par excellence), what has come to be called culture is actually "a multiply authored invention, a historical formation, an enactment, a political construct, a shifting paradox, an ongoing translation, an emblem, a trademark, a nonconsensual negotiation of contrastive identity, and more" (Boon 1990, ix). In the Portuguese Settlement, costumes, music, and dance form a bridge connecting past and present. As time and space collapse, the Settlement-as-historical-monument and the Settlement-as-housing-estate momentarily converge and become one. But the collision between real and imaginary worlds hides another inherent paradox: the past so joyously celebrated is a past that never existed. The cultural show becomes a crucible in which disparate elements meet, mingle, and together forge a new synthesis. Disguised as a representation of the "authentic," the cultural show effectively becomes an "arena of hybridization," a forum in which history is reframed, recontextualized, and—effectively—rewritten or even invented (Aggarwal 1996).

By exploring the cultural show itself, it is possible to show how this process works—how what appears to represent "authentic" tradition actually functions as an arena of hybridization. To do this, I have chosen to focus on a single performance in detail, a performance given in conjunction with Malacca Tourism Week, the annual citywide cultural festival inaugurated in 1990 and sponsored by the Malacca State Economic Development Corporation (SEDC).[1] As the well-publicized grand finale of Malacca Tourism Week 1991, this particular performance was more elaborate than an ordinary cultural show: in addition to the regular medley of dances and songs, it included a half-hour narrative "wedding scene."[2] Wedding scenes are generally only performed in the Settlement on the grandest occasions, for they are complex and relatively expensive to stage. In addition to the regular complement of musicians and dancers, a full-blown wedding scene requires at least eight extra performers and a narrator, special costumes and stage props (including wine and a wedding cake), and a large stage. Extra rehearsals must be arranged in advance and, on the day of the performance itself, extra time is needed for dressing and applying makeup (especially in the case of the "bride"). Furthermore, the inclusion of a long narrative episode is generally not practical because cultural shows are most commonly presented as floorshows in hotel restaurants, banquet halls, or shopping malls to entertain people simultaneously engaged in other activities. Nevertheless, both Rancho Folclorico San Pedro and Tropa de Malaca perform wedding scenes from time to time.

Thus, although not entirely typical of the cultural show as a genre, the particular performance under discussion is significant because it illustrates the way Settlement residents choose to represent themselves on special occasions—it is, in effect, the story they tell about themselves.[3] Given the most prestigious time slot of the citywide festival (the final Saturday night), Settlement residents chose to stage neither a generic cultural show nor what the official festival flier, produced by the Malacca Tourist Information Center, optimistically called "a 16th Century Portuguese wedding." Instead, they juxtaposed an abbreviated cultural show with a full-blown wedding scene, the former reflecting their imported Portuguese "tradition" and the latter, their indigenous, racially mixed Eurasian roots. The hybrid nature of their roots was further emphasized by the particular portion of the wedding celebration they chose to reenact: instead of selecting the most distinctly European element, the Catholic church ceremony, they re-created the bridal procession, effectively linking Settlement wedding practices with those of neighboring communities.[4] Thus, in the process of performance, Settlement residents have unconsciously constructed a perfect metaphor for their community, transforming costumes, music, and dance into crucial markers that illuminate the community's imagined and actual pasts.

This particular performance (transcribed in its entirety below) was given in the Portuguese Square on Saturday, June 1, 1991 by an enlarged Rancho Folclorico San Pedro. It was recorded by three assistants, who worked independently while I performed on stage: Sebastian de Silva ran the video camera, Yong Kok Chong took photographs, and an obliging SEDC sound engineer patched my tape recorder into the main sound system. For the sake of clarity, I have presented the transcription in three parallel columns—commentary, action, and narration—marking each significant event along a continuous timeline. Both Joe Lazaroo and his father George Bosco Lazaroo spoke in English; I have transcribed their words verbatim.

The Performance: Portuguese Settlement, Malacca, Saturday June 1, 1991

Time	Commentary (from field notes)	Action	Narration
0.00	It's about 8 P.M. and the Portuguese Square is already overflowing. The Saturday night crowd is larger than usual because of Malacca Tourism Week. Visitors from all over the world are eating and drinking as they wait for the entertainment to begin. The restaurants are all doing a roaring trade.	The musicians and dancers gather in the archway of the Portuguese Square. When they are ready, they line up behind the Rancho Folclorico San Pedro flag (an adaptation of the Portuguese flag), held by a small boy and girl from the junior dance group.	
0.55	The cumulative chatter of the crowd abates somewhat as the visitors turn their attention to the proceedings.	A female Malaysian-Chinese emcee representing the SEDC introduces the event.	
2.07	SEDC stagehands have decorated the stage with multicolored blinking lights. At the rear of the stage is a small dais on which two ornate white metal chairs have been placed. There is a white wooden screen behind the chairs with a mirror hanging at its center. To each side of the central chairs is a pair of smaller (but otherwise identical) chairs.	The musicians strike up the traditional Portuguese wedding march and the entire group processes from the archway into the Square—first the flag bearers, then the musicians, and finally the dancers in pairs. They march toward the raised concrete stage set against the sea wall.	
2.27	There are five musicians, from right to left: Basil Bournaparte (bass drum), Joe Bosco Lazaroo (guitar), Jerry Fernandis (accordion), Cypriano F. "Sub" da Costa (guitar), and myself (accordion). The men are wearing knee-length maroon pants with long white socks, light green shirts, black vests, and green *karpusu* (hats that look like woollen nightcaps) with red pom poms. I'm wearing an old dance costume (black skirt and vest with sequined edgings, white embroidered blouse, and red headscarf).	The musicians climb on to the stage, take their places stage right, and adjust their microphones. The dancers cluster in small groups on the ground to the right of the stage.	Joe Bosco Lazaroo (Joe): Good evening ladies and gentlemen and welcome to the Portuguese Settlement where Rancho Folclorico Português San Pedro will entertain you with Portuguese songs and dances from the various parts of Portugal. First, ladies and gentlemen, we going to sing and dance for you and then, to make your day a happy day, we're going to bring you up here and we going to make you dance to enjoy yourselves with us in this beautiful Portuguese Settlement.

(continued)

Time	Commentary (from field notes)	Action	Narration
3.01	The girls are wearing new dance costumes, red skirts and vests, white blouses, and red headscarves. The boys are wearing black pants with red sashes around their waists, white shirts, long-sleeved black jackets with white buttons, and black hats.	Four pairs of dancers run on to the stage as the music starts.	Joe: And the first dance is called "Ao nos' Algarve," and this type of dance comes from the south of Portugal, in the district of Algarve.
3.12	A mostly circular dance, this is RFSP's standard opening number.	Dance: "Ao nossa Algarve."	(See example 5 on p. 168.)
5.26	Changes of personnel between dances are very smooth. Although the senior dancers don't know exactly which dances Joe will call on the night, they know who dances in what and the order in which the dances are likely to appear.	The dancers leave the stage. Three couples return for the next dance.	Joe: Thank you very much. That was "Ao nos' Algarve," from the south of Portugal. Now, ladies and gentlemen, let me take you to the north of Portugal, in a place called Minho, where the Portuguese specializes in *viras* and we have "Vira di Sta. Marta."
5.47	Although there are words to this dance, Joe performs it instrumentally with Jerry leading on accordion. Alternating between line formations and the twirling of partners, this is RFSP's standard second dance.	Dance (instrumental): "Vira di Sta. Marta." The dance has an abrupt ending; after the final twirl, the girls sit on the bended knees of their male partners, who each have one arm raised as they shout "olé."	(See example 6 on p. 169.)
7.06	Joe always intersperses dances with songs, partly for variety and partly to rest the dancers. The first song (either "Cochicho da menina" or "April in Portugal") generally occurs after two dances. Though he has an extensive song repertory, Joe is relatively consistent in his choices during cultural shows for the sake of his accompanying musicians. Joe pronounces this title "Kusishu."	The dancers leave the stage as Joe starts to speak.	Joe: That was "Vira di Sta. Marta" from the north of Portugal. On a beautiful festive night, ladies and gentlemen, you find young girls beautifully dressed and walking along the road . . . and then you find young men sitting around somewhere, smiling at the girls and whistling at the girls, something like [does a catcall whistle]—I'm sure you heard this type of whistle before. "Whistling at the Girls," "Cochicho da menina."

7.40	The dancers rest and watch from off stage.	Song: "Cochicho da menina." Joe sings with Sub providing the harmonies.	
9.36	After standard opening numbers, the middle order of the program is variable. Joe calls dances depending on his mood and on the length of the show. The dancers need to stay alert and listen to his verbal cues.	Two pairs of dancers climb up to the stage as Joe is making the introduction.	Joe: Thank you very much! That was "Whistling at the Girls," "Cochicho da menina." And now, ladies and gentlemen, the favorite dance of the Portuguese: "O Malhão."
9.54	The first half of this dance comprises square and crossing patterns; the second half emphasizes line formations.	Dance: "O Malhão." [Unlike the older versions performed by other groups, Joe's has two distinct halves. After the first half, a sudden modulation from C major to F major leads into the standard second section.]	(See example 7 on pp. 170–71.)
11.51	Both these dances are performed by other groups, but Joe is the only one who strings them together as a medley.	The dancers leave the stage as Joe starts to speak. Three couples return for the next dance.	Joe: That was the most famous dance of the Portugal, "O Malhão." And now we have a medley of two dances and it's called "Camacha" and "Regadinho." "Camacha" is a farmers' dance. The mother asks the son to water the plants and the son says, "why should I water the plants when my love is waiting for me on the other side of the garden?" And "Regadinho" is a lovers' dance.
12.21	"Camacha" [pronounced "Kamasha"] employs mostly circular patterns broken by individual couples twirling. In "Regadinho" [pronounced "Regadinyo"] the couples alternate between turning in pairs and promenading in a circular formation.	Dance: "Camacha." Segues straight into: Dance: "Regadinho."	(See example 8 on p. 171.) (See example 9 on p. 172.)

(continued)

Time	Commentary (from field notes)	Action	Narration
15.01	The junior girls are wearing the same black dance costumes as myself; the junior boys are wearing black vests instead of jackets and have no hats. "Tiru Liru Liru" is Joe's standard penultimate dance. While the other groups perform it as a regular dance, Joe uses it as a vehicle to encourage audience participation and as a warm up to his final number.	The dancers leave the stage as Joe starts to speak. Six couples, including some of the junior dancers, take their places on stage. They line up in two blocks of three couples each. Within each block, partners face each other and neighbors alternate (boy-girl-boy facing girl-boy-girl).	Joe: That was a medley of two dances "Camacha" and "Regadinho." Well, ladies and gentlemen, like I said in the beginning that we will try to make you dance. You watch this dance carefully; it's called "Tiru Liru Liru." It says, "let's go up, let's go down, together we dance." So, ladies and gentlemen, you put on dancing shoes and the dancers will come down and bring you up here and you going to enjoy yourselves—thousands did it before, tonight is your lucky night and we will see that you do it. You watch this dance, we only going to do it once. Only once. Watch this dance carefully and then we're going to bring you up. . . . "Tiru Liru Liru."
16.01	This is a simple line dance comprising mostly hand motions and turning on the spot.	Dance: "Tiru Liru Liru."	(See example 10 on p. 172.)
17.05	With beer flowing at all the restaurants, there is no problem finding volunteers from the audience.	The dancers leave the stage and mingle with the audience, asking for dance partners.	Joe: OK, ladies and gentlemen, the dancers are coming down and they're going to bring you up here so that you can say to your friends back home, I did Portuguese dance in the Portuguese Settlement, Malacca.
17.26	Although it is hard to get a precise sense of where the volunteers come from, they are mostly Western or Chinese (probably Singaporean). Settlement residents who happen to be in the Square are often invited by the shyer dancers.	The stage gradually fills as each senior and junior dancer brings up a partner of the opposite sex.	Joe: Come on, ladies and gentlemen, thousands did it before. Like I said, tonight is your lucky night. I see one couple, two couples, three couples—coming up—come on, four couples. Ladies and gentlemen, come on! You are here to enjoy yourselves during this Tourism Week.

18.16	The stage is now crowded. Some volunteers wave at their friends and receive cheers of encouragement from the floor, others look around with bemused expressions on their faces.	The dancers line their new partners up into rows, which observe the same boy-girl-boy pattern. Each volunteer thus faces a member of the dance group and has dancers of the opposite sex on either side.	Joe: Actually, ladies and gentlemen, we don't have to teach you this dance. It's so simple that you only have to follow your own partners in front of you and you can do it right. Are you ready? Watch the partners in front of you.
18.47	The dance is easy, but it still causes much hilarity among the audience, especially when the volunteers have to turn around.	Dance: "Tiru Liru Liru." The volunteers imitate the movements of their partners or their neighbors.	
19.40		The dancers and the tourists all leave the stage.	Joe: Look at that—beautiful dancers! Come on, let's give them a big, big hand, ladies and gentlemen, come on. Beautiful to see so many of them up here.
19.57	"Baile de Roda" is the usual last dance of the standard RFSP show. The main portion of the dance is the fastest and most virtuosic circular dance of their repertory. Although the dance can be the finale per se, Joe generally turns the final chorus into a repetitive vamp to provide another opportunity for audience participation.	Four couples climb on to the stage as Joe is making the introduction.	Joe: The next dance is called "Baile de Roda." It's a fast little dance, and ladies and gentlemen, this dance is not complete if you don't dance with them. We know you're professional dancers, so we're not going to teach you this dance. What the dancers are going to do is they going down and they going to pull you up and we're going to dance from here to the car park and back. Well, we try. If we cannot, at least we try. "Baile de Roda."
20.36		Dance: "Baile de Roda." Toward the end of the dance, the boys lift the girls up to their shoulders and continue turning in a circle. As the dance ends, the musicians repeat the chorus and the dancers leave the stage.	(See example 11 on p. 173.)
23.10	All dancers, senior and junior, are mobilized for this last dance.	The chorus continues. Sub takes over the singing as Joe encourages the audience. The dancers pick partners from the crowd.	Joe: OK, ladies and gentlemen, the dancers are coming down for you. . . . .

(continued)

Time	Commentary (from field notes)	Action	Narration
23.22	The conga-like line is led by Joe's daughter, Elaine, and her partner, a blond male European.	The chorus continues. Dancers, their partners, and even enthusiastic pairs of audience members join the line that criss-crosses the Square. Finally, Elaine leads the line up to the stage. She and her partner form an arch, through which the other dancers pass. The line continues to weave around the stage until Joe's cue.	Joe: Come on, make it your night, come on. . . .
25.02	Locals have no problem switching since *branyo* steps are the same as those of *joget*: the foreigners improvise.	At the end of the chorus, Basil hammers out the *branyo* rhythm on bass drum and the musicians segue into "Jinkly Nona."	Joe: And now for the traditional *branyo*, ladies and gentlemen. . . .
25.13		*Branyo*: "Jinkly Nona." Sub sings the verses, Joe leads the choruses.	
26.30	[Both video and audio tapes fade out during the transition. To compensate for this hiatus, I have added 5 minutes to all subsequent timings.]	The dancers and their partners applaud each other as they leave the stage.	Joe: Well look at that, ladies and gentlemen, how they enjoy themselves. At least they can say to their friends back home, we did Portuguese dances in this beautiful Portuguese Settlement, Malacca. Give us only three minutes, ladies and gentlemen, and we will get on with the traditional Portuguese wedding.
32.43	A small table with a white lace cloth and a large two-layer white wedding cake have been placed in front of the two large chairs. A mitre-shaped decoration (*kronchi*) made from silver foil has been hung over the center of the mirror behind the chairs. A symbol of purity, *kronchis* are hung over the front door (to announce that a household is involved in a wedding) and over the door to the bridal suite (to bless the bridal couple). The musicians, still at stage left, adjust microphones and chat as they wait.		George Bosco Lazaroo (Bosco): Imagine to yourselves that you are cordially invited to this Portuguese wedding. As the music is being played, please welcome the entourage with a rousing, standing ovation. The entourage is composed of the bride and bridegroom, the man sponsor, and the lady sponsor. Ladies and gentlemen, the wedding ceremony; it is the moment you are waiting for. The traditional music gives flavor to the occasion, and all eyes are focused on the married couple.

33.36	The procession comprises bride (Sharon Fanwell), groom (Christopher de Mello), *kumadri* (Theresa da Costa), and *kumpadri* (Joe "Bomba" Lazaroo). (The nickname *bomba*, "fireman," refers to his former job and avoids confusion with the other Joe Lazaroo, Joe Bosco.) Sharon and 'Pher are both RFSP dancers; Uncle Joe "Bomba" plays tambourine with the group.	Music: the Portuguese wedding march. This continues to be played softly in the background throughout the commentary. The tourists applaud the bride (on the left) and the groom (on the right) as they lead the procession through the archway into the Square. They are followed by two other couples, the *kumadri* and *kumpadri*, and the bridesmaid and best man.	Bosco: Here they are, give them a big, big hand. . . .
33.55	The groom is wearing a white suit with a black hat; the *kumpadri* wears a dark suit. Bosco describes the bride's outfit himself. In addition, she has on an elaborate headdress and an ornate necklace. The *kumadri* is wearing a traditional formal dress—a colorful long blouse (called *kebaya kompridu* in Kristang or *baju kurung* in Malay) over a matching long skirt. The blouse is fastened by three golden pins (called *kerungsang*).	Music: the Portuguese wedding march. The procession moves slowly through the Square.	Bosco: The bridegroom in full suit handles his charming wife. She is dressed in immaculate white, which is the *kebaya* and *sáia* and carrying in her hand is a bouquet of beautiful white flowers. [Pause.] They both smile to the guests as they slowly, step by step, walk and stops in front of the stage.
35.29	The bridesmaid (Valerie Plera) is wearing a *kebaya kompridu* and the best man (Walter Nathan), a dark blue suit. Both Valerie and Walter are regular RFSP dancers. The brooch, which other sources say should be pinned to the bride's dress, is also called *kronchi*. Like the hanging ornament, it symbolizes virginity.	Music: the Portuguese wedding march. The bridal party pauses half way between the archway and the left side of the Square. They are met by the bridesmaid and best man, who approach them carrying a tray and a pin/brooch. After placing the brooch on the bride's head, they shake hands with and back away from the bridal couple.	Bosco: Ladies and gentlemen, the wedding ceremony proper begins here. [Pause.] You will witness the bridesmaid, known as—in Portuguese—as *mara kronchi femi* is accompanied by the best man, known as the *mara kronchi machu*. He carries the tray on which is a valuable pin. They both approach the married couple. The bride beside her bends slowly, slightly forward, and the *mara kronchi femi* takes the pin, which is known as the *kronchi*, places this on the bride's head. They both congratulate the married couple. This *kronchi* is a symbol of purity.

(continued)

Time	Commentary (from field notes)	Action	Narration
36.32	Traditionally the bridal couple are received by their parents and relatives at the bride's house. In this case, there is only one set of "parents" in the receiving party: Norman de Mello and Theodora Lazaroo (better known as "Aunty Girl"). Uncle Norman is wearing a white suit and Aunty Girl is wearing a colorful *kebaya kompridu*.	Music: the Portuguese wedding march. 'Pher, the groom, follows Bosco's directions.	Bosco: The bridegroom takes leave from his bride, moves a few steps forward, takes off his hat, and as a mark of respect, graciously bows to the parents, then turns round and bows to his beloved wife, who curtseys with a loving smile. He then turns round again to the invited guests, and bows to them to show the gratitude and appreciate their attendance to his wedding. He returns and joins his anxious wife who has been left lonely for a short while, handles her gently, and moves forward with the entourage following.
37.52		Music: the Portuguese wedding march. The bridesmaid and best man walk backward as they sprinkle water and flowers over the bridal couple. They lead the way up to the stage.	Bosco: The couple approaches the parents who stand at the door, eagerly awaiting their arrival. . . . they wish them and kisses the hands, the Portuguese custom and it is a sign of respect and gratitude. [Pause.] Music goes on and as they enter the house, the bridesmaid throws scented flowers and the best man, holding a *stroyi*, which is a silver receptacle filled with scented water, sprinkles on the bride and bridegroom all the way till they are in the house.
39.19		Music: the Portuguese wedding march.	Bosco: In the house, you will observe that there is a mirror placed behind the bride. Her head-dress is reflected on the mirror for the guests to admire the unique and valuable ornament.
39.41	The characters are seated as follows (left to right from the audience perspective): Uncle Norman (father), Uncle Joe "Bomba" (*kumpadri*), 'Pher (groom), Sharon (bride), Aunty Theresa (*kumadri*), Aunty Girl (mother).	The music stops. The bride and groom sit down on the two central chairs. They are flanked by the sponsors and parents, who take the smaller chairs (men are seated stage right, women stage left).	Bosco: The bride and bridegroom sit in juxtaposition. Next to the bride sits the lady sponsor and beside the bridegroom is the man sponsor. These two personalities are very important witnesses of the marriage. The parents, the best man, and the bridesmaid sit in their proper places. Joy and happiness personified can be seen on their faces. It is indeed an auspicious day.

40.43	The "guests" chairs are placed stage left at right angles to the wedding party. There are two rows of four or five chairs each.	The dancers bring tourists up to the stage to shake hands with the bridal couple, groom first and then the bride. The dancers then lead the "guests" to their seats.	Bosco: The Portuguese dancers, dressed in beautiful multicolored costumes, and with the latest Hollywood makeup on their faces, blended with smiles, portrays typical Portuguese dances from one of the hamlets in Portugal. They will feel jealous and I hope not. These dancers at this point will personally invite a few guests from the floor to come up to the stage to congratulate the married couple and sit down on the seats provided for them.
41.43		There is a long silence as the tourist guests line up to shake hands with the bride and groom.	Bosco: The invited guests will congratulate the bride and the bridegroom. And they will take their seats on the chairs provided.
43.36	The Portuguese costumes of the dancers contrast sharply with the traditional clothes and suits of the wedding party. The three assistants are all senior dancers.	The dancers assist with the proceedings: Elaine Lazaroo and Juana Lai each take a layer of cake to be cut and Anthony Lazaroo removes the table. Tourists crowd in front of the stage to take pictures.	Bosco: The wedding cake is the next center of attraction. It is ready to be cut. The bride and bridegroom stand before this beautifully decorated wedding cake. The bridegroom places his hand on the bride's hand, presses the knife on the decorated cake, especially prepared for the occasion. The married couple take their seats and cake and wine will be served to the couple, family, and invited guests on the stage.
44.46	Members of the bridal party remain seated as they listen to the music.	Song: "Vira di Bairu Português." The bridesmaid distributes napkins, first to the tourist guests at the side of the stage, then to the bridal party.	(See example 12 on p. 174.)
46.48	This song is one of Joe's own compositions. It is the only piece of music heard so far, except for the *branyo* tune "Jinkly Nona" and possibly the wedding march, that is indigenous to the Settlement.	The music stops.	Joe: That was the dance of the people of the Portuguese Settlement, "Vira di Bairu Português."
47.57	The musicians debate what to play next and settle on an Iberian-sounding waltz from Jerry's repertoire. We all follow his lead as best we can.	The bridesmaid and best man serve cake and wine to the bridal party and to the tourist guests. Music: instrumental waltz led by Jerry Fernandis on accordion.	

(continued)

Time	Commentary (from field notes)	Action	Narration
48.55		Music: the waltz continues softly. The best man refills the glasses of the tourist guests.	Bosco: Please hold on to your glasses.
50.17		The music stops. One of the musicians hands the *kumpadri*, Joe "Bomba," a microphone.	Bosco: The man sponsor, known in Portuguese, the *kumpadri*, gives a toast to the married couple in Portuguese language.
50.27	Bosco's simultaneous translation overlaps and sometimes obscures the words of the *kumpadri*'s Kristang toast.	Uncle Joe "Bomba" takes the microphone and raises his glass to give a toast in Kristang. All members of the bridal party stand and raise their glasses toward the bride and groom.	Joe "Bomba" and [Bosco]: *Siara, sioras* [Ladies and gentlemen] *isi teng kazamintu* [this is a toast to the married couple] *isi teng saude di noiba ku noibu. Ozendia olotu ja fica kambradu* [I am happy to see such a large crowd of friends] *yo bong poku allegra ki yo ja ola tantu nossa primo primos ja beng attinda na isi kazamintu* [many of my relatives are here too]. *Nos bota riba nossa kopu* [Lift your glasses and let us drink to the] *da saude ku noiba ku noibu* [good health and prosperity] . . . unclear . . . *saude. Saude noiba ku noibu.* [Let's drink to the health and prosperity of the married couple. Enjoy yourselves with the cake and wine].
51.27		The bride and groom finally eat their cake. Following Bosco's directions, the tourist guests also eat and chat among themselves.	Bosco: At this stage, the music perfumes the air while the invited guests on the stage converse freely and partake of the delicious wedding cake ordered especially for this grand function. Soft music is being played.
52.04	This is not one of the songs Joe regularly uses in cultural shows, so I don't know it well. Sub leans over and calls out the chords as we play.	The bridesmaid and best man serve more cake and wine to the tourist guests. Music: instrumental version of "Lisboa Antiga," led by Jerry Fernandis on accordion.	

53.51	The *branyo* is, indeed, the traditional dance of the Portuguese Settlement and a favorite feature at any wedding or festive occasion. Whether it is 400 years old and/or of Portuguese origin as Bosco would have us believe, is debatable.	The dancers, senior and junior, return to the stage and invite the tourist guests to join them in the *branyo*.	Joe "Bomba" and [Bosco]: *Siara, sioras* [The *kumpadri* announces, Ladies and gentlemen] *Considra* [Take it] *agora nus ja kumi bebe chegar* [that we have enjoyed ourselves] *oras di allegria mesti chegar* [now the time has come for us to make merry] *beng nus kada kuái, toma nus sapatineros; beng nus allegra, nus bala, bersu branyo* [to be happy and gay. Select your partners and dance the 400-years-old Portuguese traditional *branyo* to the rhythm of the accordion, the guitar, and the drum. Please don't be shy. Smile and dance, dance, dance]. *Siara, sioras.* . . .
54.42		Music: *branyo* tune "Jinkly Nona." Sub sings the verses, Joe leads the chorus. The bride, groom, wedding party, and the tourist guests rise, move to the center of the stage and begin to dance the local *branyo*.	
56.11	The transition from "Jinkly Nona" to "Bong Bong Fila" is managed so skillfully, no one misses a step. Both melodies draw upon the same body of stock quatrains.	The musicians segue straight into a second *branyo* tune, "Bong Bong Fila"; this time, Joe sings the verses.	
57.51		The tourist guests and the dancers gradually leave the stage during Bosco's closing remarks.	Bosco: Ladies and gentlemen, we have come to the end of *kazamintu di portugês*, the Portuguese wedding ceremony of bygone days, which is a night to remember. You have enjoyed the dance, you have enjoyed the show, a feast for your eyes. The narrator, George Bosco Lazaroo, signs off and wishes you, good people of Malacca and those tourists from far off lands, a very good night, sweet dreams as you throw yourselves into the arms of Morpheus, and God bless you and your family.

(continued)

Time	Commentary (from field notes)	Action	Narration
58.41	This is the standard closing formula for RFSP shows. The march tune is repeated while dancers and musicians all take their bows.	Music: closing march. The members of the wedding party come forward, pause for photographs, then bow and leave the stage. Next, the RFSP dancers return, form two lines and take their bows (girls first, then boys). Finally, the musicians come forward in a row and bow, still playing as they leave the stage.	Bosco: Thank you ladies and gentlemen, friends and all, who attending the wedding of the year.
58.51		Music: closing march, fading as musicians approach the archway.	SEDC emcee: Ladies and gentlemen, let's give our Rancho Folclorico San Pedro Cultural Show an appreciation by giving them a big hand. Yes, thank you ladies and gentlemen, thank you for your clap.
59.39	Some of the tourists begin to make their way back to their waiting buses; others relax and continue to enjoy their food and drink. Once the cultural show is over, the regular nightly entertainment begins as Chico de Costa (guitar) and his cousin, John (keyboards), sing golden oldies until the wee hours of the morning.	Music stops as the musicians leave the Square.	SEDC emcee: One more time, a big hand for the San Pedro cultural troupe. Thank you very much. Ladies and gentlemen, with this we close off the event for the evening. I sincerely hope you have enjoyed yourselves and had a very entertaining evening. We have some announcements here. Tomorrow evening we'll be having a variety of cultural dances here performed by the various local cultural groups. . . .
60.12	[Audio tape fades out here]		

Reading the Performance

As can be seen from the transcription, the performance falls into two parts, roughly equal in terms of duration but otherwise clearly distinct. Taken together, they appear to reflect neatly the competing faces of the Settlement-as-historical-monument and the Settlement-as-housing-estate. At first sight, the cultural show typifies the imported tradition-that-never-was of the former, while the latter is evoked by a dramatized segment of an old-time Eurasian wedding, a reconstructed part of traditional Settlement life that is no longer actually practiced. Closer examination shows, however, that in the glare of the spotlights, there is seepage between worlds, causing bizarre and improbable juxtapositions.

The performance begins with an abbreviated version of a typical Rancho Folclorico San Pedro cultural show, a continuous medley of dances with a single song providing momentary relief for the dancers (see fig. 12).[5] Throughout this part of the show, Joe Lazaroo is clearly the dominant performer, the only one who stands out as a distinct—albeit nameless—personality. He functions as his own emcee: deciding what to sing and dance, introducing each number, and addressing the audience directly. Although few outsiders would notice, Joe's running commentary is not as spontaneous as it sounds; the introductions and jokes have been honed over many years and are reused at each new performance. The predictability of his patter actually serves a practical function—that of

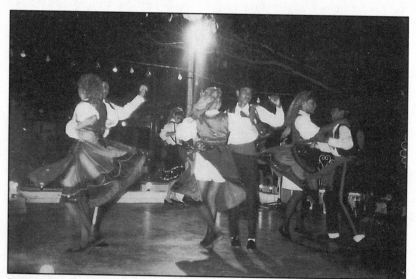

Figure 12 Rancho Folclorico San Pedro performing in first half of the wedding scene. Photograph by Yong Kok Chong

cuing the other musicians and the dancers. As soon as he utters the first words of his introduction, the designated dancers return to the stage and smoothly assume their opening formation while the musicians strum the opening chords quietly in the background. Despite appearances, there are two significant departures from normal routine: the opening march and the stage setting. On the rare occasions that Rancho Folclorico San Pedro performances begin with a procession, the musical accompaniment is not the "Portuguese wedding march" but the nameless march also used for final bows. On this special occasion, however, the wedding march becomes a frame, linking the "Portuguese" cultural dance show with the indigenous wedding scene, thus unifying the two disparate halves of the performance. The wedding scene set (dais, chairs, wooden screen, and mirror) serves a similar unifying function. Displacing the musicians from their usual upstage center location to a peripheral position upstage right, the empty set links the dancers to the wedding celebration, making them part of action yet to unfold.

The dynamics of the performance change when the wedding scene begins. No longer emcee and dominant personality, Joe is relegated to the secondary role of a hired musician playing background music.[6] His father, George Bosco Lazaroo, takes control of the performance, positioning his microphone upstage left and using the set to separate himself from Joe and the other musicians. Unlike Joe's first-half persona, Bosco stands outside the action. He functions not as a leader who actively determines the proceedings while maintaining an unmediated relationship with the audience, but as a commentator who describes and explains the unfolding action, barely looking at the audience as he watches the progress of the actors and reads from a prepared script.[7] Once again, however, there is an overlap as elements from the first half of the performance impinge upon the second half. This time the seepage between worlds is human: without changing their costumes, the "Portuguese" musicians and dancers of Rancho Folclorico San Pedro return to the stage and become participants in the old-time Settlement wedding.

It quickly becomes clear, then, that the two seemingly disparate halves of the performance are actually linked in subtle ways to form a complex synthesis. Individual elements—such as dress, music, dance, and the participants themselves—are fused to create a richly textured story that is neither historically accurate nor a representation of present-day practice. And yet, the end result, regardless of its historical veracity, is the story residents of the Portuguese Settlement tell about themselves.

As such, it is worth examining closely to find out exactly what it is they say.

Dress

Dress is the most potent visual element of this synthesis. Although observers may be unaware of the conflicting messages conveyed by the costumes, it is obvious that different types of costume are used (in increasingly mixed combinations) over the course of the performance. This diversity is not apparent at the outset, however; costumes used during the cultural show are relatively homogeneous. Subsets of Rancho Folclorico San Pedro—musicians, senior female and senior male dancers, junior female and junior male dancers—wear different costumes, but all look equally "Portuguese." Conforming to familiar stereotypes of Portuguese dress and placed within the legitimizing frame of the cultural show, the authenticity of RFSP costumes is not questioned. Most of the costumes are, in Bruner's terms, "credible and convincing": locally made, some, like the senior boys' black jackets with their distinctive white buttons, are copied from book illustrations (in this case, from the Minho region), while others are locally designed. The only items that could perhaps be seen as original and "the real thing" are the green and red *karpusu* hats worn by the musicians, which were sent to Malacca as gifts from Portugal—modern, not sixteenth-century Portugal. Of course, expecting to see traditional costumes on display at cultural shows, most observers assume that the costumes seen on stage are the traditional dress of the people wearing them.

This assumption is challenged as soon as the second half of the performance begins. Although the musicians remain on stage in their Portuguese costumes, the members of the wedding procession are dressed quite differently. The men of the cast—groom, *kumpadri* (male sponsor), best man, and father—wear Western suits and ties while the *kumadri* (female sponsor), bridesmaid, and mother wear colorful three-quarter-length blouses *(kebaya kompridu)* fastened by three gold pins *(kerungsang)* and worn over long skirts *(sáia)*. Looking more Malay than any costume seen so far, *kebaya kompridu* is the traditional formal dress of Settlement women (see fig. 13). Even the name reflects its hybrid origin: *kebaya* is Malay for "blouse," but *kompridu* is Kristang for "long." Although the formal *kebaya kompridu* is rarely worn today, many older women still wear *sarong kebaya*—short blouses over long Malay-style sarongs—around the Settlement (see fig. 14). The term *sáia kebaya* used by Bosco in his narra-

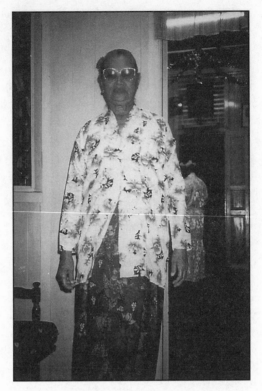

Figure 13   Theodora Lazaroo, the wedding scene mother
of the bride, in formal *kebaya kompridu.*

tion again shows hybrid influence, mixing Kristang (*sáia,* "skirt") with
Malay (*kebaya,* "blouse").

The bride wears similar dress—a white silk *kebaya* and *sáia* with an
elaborate golden headdress and ornate necklace (see fig. 15). The Malay
influence on the bride's dress is clear if we compare it to one used in a
Malay wedding scene performance (see fig. 16). While the brides are
dressed alike, the clothes worn by the two grooms point to different
worlds: one Western, the other Malay. In the Settlement performance,
this sartorial difference is a crucial reminder of a distant mixed-race past.
As explained by Settlement resident, Patrick de Silva:

> Marriages were basically between Portuguese men and Malay damsels. In
> the absence of Portuguese families, it is obvious that marriage arrangements
> were made by the bride's family. Hence, the bride's costume followed local
> traditions. Considering the norms of those times, no parent would be naive
> as to discard traditions, let alone adopt a foreign one. With this tradition

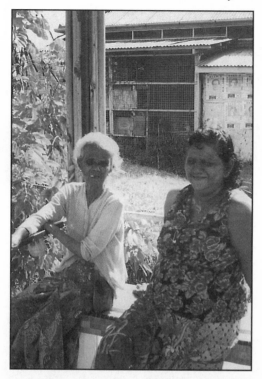

Figure 14 Two Settlement women in everyday
sarong kebaya (Aunty Philomena and Theresa de Costa).

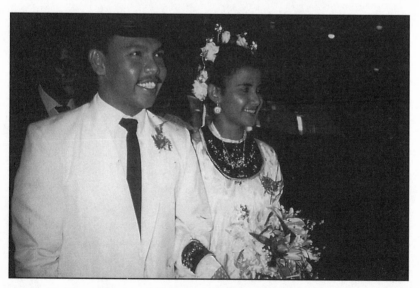

Figure 15 The wedding scene bride and groom (Christopher de Mello and Sharon Fanwell).
Photograph by Yong Kok Chong

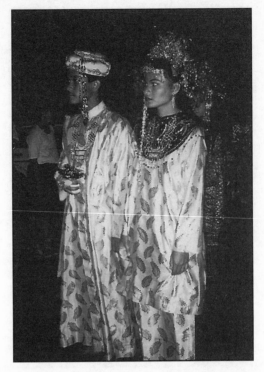

Figure 16   Malay wedding scene bride and groom.

being handed down from mother to daughter, it finally became part and parcel of the local-born Portuguese tradition in Malacca, and is still being kept alive to a lesser extent. (de Silva 1987, 84)

As the bridal party processes through the Square, another bridge between past and present is created. While there is a measure of romanticization—conjuring up the ghosts of handsome Portuguese *fidalgos* and their beautiful local brides—there is also a certain historical truth: the generic Western suits and Malay dresses powerfully highlight the community's mixed-race Eurasian (though not necessarily Portuguese)[8] past, while the Malay-style procession emphasizes the hybridity of its more recent past. The moment the bride, groom, and their retinue climb onto the stage, however, they enter the world of the imagined. Once again, the stage becomes a crucible, fusing disparate worlds into an original synthesis. Temporal and spatial distances collapse as members of the bridal party take their seats on the wedding-scene set and Rancho Folclorico San Pedro dancers return to the stage. The dancers in their Portuguese costumes, the imaginary descendants of D'Albuquerque, bring members of the audience up to the stage to congratulate the bride and groom. In the process, a third world is absorbed unwittingly into the synthesis: spectators from the audience are transformed into wedding guests and become part of the performance.

One person on stage remains aloof. The narrator, George Bosco Lazaroo, stands alone, upstage left, next to the steps that performers use to reach the stage, effectively marking the intersection between real and imagined worlds. This spatial separation is reinforced sartorially: he is the only person on stage (except, of course, for the tourist guests) not "dressed up." The other performers are all wearing special costumes of one sort or another, whether the Portuguese costumes of the RFSP musicians and dancers, the dress suits of the male wedding scene characters, or the formal *kebaya kompridu* of the female characters. But Bosco, standing outside the action, wears what he always wears, the traditional everyday dress of older Settlement men: a thin, white short-sleeved t-shirt and faded blue and white striped pajama-like trousers *(jempata)* tied with a rope string around the middle. A Settlement resident's casual remark—"the Malays call this *baju melayu* (Malay: "Malay dress"), but it's actually Portuguese costume"—is telling, for it emphasizes the hybridity of this informal dress. In the everyday world of the Settlement-as-housing-estate, then, the men (and their clothes) are no longer European; they are just as racially mixed as the women.

Music and Dance

The synthesis forged in the Portuguese Square, the story Settlement residents tell about themselves, becomes even richer and more complex when we take into account two other equally important elements of the performance: music and dance. During the first half hour, the combination of stereotypically Portuguese costumes and the sanctioned forum of the cultural show suggests that we are about to witness (in Joe Lazaroo's own words) "Portuguese songs and dances from the various parts of Portugal." Again, the frame legitimizes the contents, and the authenticity of Rancho Folclorico San Pedro's repertoire goes unquestioned. The unspoken implication—that these particular songs and dances have been preserved by Settlement residents over many generations—becomes another bridge between past and present. This time, dress disguises difference: the impression of homogeneity created by costumes and context is, in fact, contested by music and dance.

At the outset, the performance appears to conform to Joe Lazaroo's initial promise. The first two dances ("Ao nosso Algarve" and "Vira di Sta. Marta") are carefully attributed to regions of Portugal well known for folkloric music and dance—Algarve and Minho, respectively.[9] Thereafter, Joe's introductions become increasingly less specific. He only associates one further dance, "O Malhão," directly with Portugal (and then only vaguely, calling it "the most famous dance of Portugal"). Of the other items on the program, "Cochicho da menina" and "Camacha" are both prefaced with brief stories, "Regadinho" is simply called a "lovers' dance," "Tiru Liru Liru" is introduced by translating a short segment of its text, and "Baile de Roda" is described only as "a fast little dance."

While it is true that all the dances and the single song originated in Portugal, not all were imported at the same time and none date back— in Malaysia, at least—to mythical Portuguese times. The opening and closing dances—"Ao nosso Algarve," "Vira di Sta. Marta," and "Baile de Roda"—are the fastest, most virtuosic items on the program. All three belong to the repertoire introduced since 1974 by Fr. Sendim and Christie Rodrigues and classified within the Settlement as "Portuguese music." Although the origin of "Regadinho" is unknown, its straightforward melody and choreography have ensured its adoption by the other groups. The RFSP version of "O Malhão" is unique in the Settlement repertoire in that it appears to juxtapose two completely different musical and choreographic versions of the dance. The virtuosic first part belongs to the Sendim-Rodrigues repertoire; half way through the dance, however, a sudden modulation from C major to F major leads into a simpler older version that has been performed in the Settlement since 1953 and is now considered "our music."[10] "Tiru Liru Liru" dates from the same period as the older version of "O Malhão": it was one of the two dances on the program for the Portuguese minister's visit in 1952.[11] No one remembers exactly when "Camacha" was introduced, but it is generally thought to be among the older pieces in the repertoire.

The bulk of the material used in this particular abbreviated cultural dance show, then, was imported at one time or another from Portugal, supporting the illusion created by the costumes.[12] Though the costumes were designed in the Settlement, they imitate Portuguese models; though the dances may well have been modified (or even reset) by choreographer Christie Rodrigues, they are based on Portuguese models. And yet, the two outermost pieces—the opening instrumental march and the closing *branyo*—contest this picture. Although neither piece is introduced by title—in fact, Joe does not mention the march at all—both the "Portuguese wedding march" and the *branyo* tune "Jinkly Nona" are crucial links to the second half of the performance.

The performance begins with Rancho Folclorico San Pedro musicians and dancers, in Portuguese costume, processing through the Square to the repeated strains of a stately march. Although there is nothing to suggest to the spectators that they are listening to a *wedding* march, the harmonic structure, steady four-square rhythm, and military bass drum accompaniment all suggest that the march is of European origin, an impression strengthened by the context (costumes and placement at the start of a Portuguese cultural dance show). This impression is challenged, however, when the march returns at the start of the second half. It is still used to accompany a procession, but the stationary on-stage musicians and the cultural group dancers are no longer part of the entourage. Instead, the participants are marked by their clothing as mixed-race Eurasians. Costume, the association with a wedding procession, and Bosco's description of the march as "traditional music [that] gives flavor to the occasion" now suggest not only that it is a wedding march but also that it is a wedding march of local rather than imported origin. This second interpretation corresponds to Settlement opinion. No one is completely sure about the history of the march, but according to Joe Lazaroo, it has been played as far back as he can remember and it originated in the Settlement (pers. comm., August 27, 1997).

Like the wedding march, the *branyo* is performed twice. The first time it occurs (at the end of the first half), it is thoroughly integrated into the cultural dance show. As the last dance, "Baile de Roda," nears completion, the dancers leave the stage and mingle with the audience. Over the continuously repeating chorus, they invite spectators to join them, form a conga-like line, and wind their way around the Square. When the dancers and their new partners finally return to the stage, Joe shouts over the repeating chorus, "And now for the traditional *branyo,* ladies and gentlemen." Basil Bournaparte gives a cue on his bass drum, and once again disparate worlds collide: the musicians segue seamlessly from their modern Portuguese dance into the old-time Settlement favorite, "Jinkly Nona"; the dancers, in their Portuguese costumes, break out of line formation, face their new partners, and begin to dance the local *branyo.* Although this is the only time Joe uses the word "traditional," the costumes and transition from "Baile de Roda" confuse the picture. Foreign tourists, who have spent the last half hour watching "Portuguese dance," have no way of knowing whether "traditional *branyo*" refers to a traditional Portuguese or a traditional Settlement dance. Domestic (Malaysian and Singaporean) members of the audience, however, instantly recognize the *branyo* for what it is: a hybrid. The Kristang lyrics may be incomprehensible to them, but the rhythm and steps of the *branyo*—unlike anything seen on stage to this point—are identical to the Malay social dance, the *joget.*

When the *branyo* is performed again at the end of the wedding scene, it is not the coda to a previous piece but an independent, unchoreographed social dance. As such it functions only secondarily as entertainment for the audience in the Square; its primary function is to entertain the onstage cast: wedding party, Portuguese dancers, and invited tourist guests. For a moment, the audience in the Square is forgotten and the musicians switch from one *branyo* melody, "Jinkly Nona," to another, "Bong bong fila," just as they would at a real wedding to prolong the social dancing. The synthesis is momentarily complete as the mythical world of D'Albuquerque, the old-time world of the Settlement, and the many worlds of the tourist guests are fused on stage. For audience members remaining in their seats, however, Bosco's introduction—"Select your partners and dance the four-hundred-years-old Portuguese traditional *branyo*"—compounds the ambiguity introduced by his son. On the one hand, he appears to say (to foreigners) that the *branyo* is a traditional Portuguese dance that is four-hundred years old. His implication—that this particular traditional Portuguese dance has been performed continuously by the Malacca community for four-hundred years—once again connects his community to mythic times. On the other hand, by emphasizing the unchanging longevity of the "Portuguese traditional dance," he denies its hybridity and implies (to the domestic audience) that the *joget,* the Malaysian national dance, is itself derived from an original Portuguese tradition.

The wedding march and *branyo,* the two local items from the otherwise imported cultural dance show, frame the domestic wedding scene. The march, repeated continuously throughout the bridal procession, ceases when the bride and groom reach the stage and take their seats on the dais. After a long silence, during which Rancho Folclorico San Pedro dancers reappear on stage bringing tourist guests to offer their congratulations and the bridesmaid and best man prepare to serve cake and wine, Joe and his musicians offer a brief musical interlude. By the time they begin their first song, the wedding party and tourist guests are all seated on stage and have become the primary audience. Significantly, instead of selecting another song from his large repertoire of Portuguese songs, Joe chooses one of his own compositions, "Vira di Bairu Portuguès." Although Joe does not acknowledge the song as his own composition, his brief aside—"that was the dance of the people of the Portuguese Settlement"—increases the expectation that, like the wedding scene itself, the interlude music is of local rather than imported origin. But once again, the stage functions as a crucible. As wine and cake are served to the wedding cast and tourist guests, the synthesis is completed. The soft background music (led by Jerry Fernandis on accordion) is not local, but imported: first, a waltz and then an instrumental version of one of Joe's favorite Portuguese songs, the Amália Rodrigues hit, "Lisboa antiga."[13]

The Players

The story Settlement residents tell about themselves is further complicated when we examine the final element in the synthesis: the players themselves. With the exception of George Bosco Lazaroo, who introduces himself by name, and Joe Lazaroo, we see musicians, dancers, and actors, not individuals. To spectators, the musicians and dancers of Rancho Folclorico San Pedro are interchangeable, distinguished only by costume. The cast of the wedding scene, in contrast, is more distinctive, because each member plays a readily identifiable role defined by familiar bounded relationships: the married couple, the parents of the bride, sponsors *(kumpadri* and *kumadri),* and peers (bridesmaid and best man). But, just as real and imagined worlds are fused on stage, so too are real and imagined human relationships. The clear-cut onstage roles are often contradicted by complex real life affiliations (as might occur in any theatrical performance) that frequently place real life relatives in unusual relationships to each other.

For example, on stage, the father of the bride is played by Norman de Mello. In real life, however, he is the father of the groom, Christopher, and also, incidentally, of Tropa de Malaca's Anne and Laura and father-in-law of Anne's husband, Gerard da Costa—himself a nephew of Theresa da Costa, the *kumadri,* and first cousin of "Sub," the guitarist. Norman de Mello was also, in his younger days, one of the members of the first Settlement dance group. Theodora Lazaroo (nicknamed "Aunty Girl") plays the mother of the bride and stage wife of Norman. Off stage, she is actually the wife of the narrator, George Bosco Lazaroo, mother of Joe Lazaroo, and grandmother of Joe's daughter and senior dancer, Elaine. Joe "Bomba" Lazaroo, who has traded his tambourine and RFSP musician's costume to play the role of *kumpadri,* is the real-life father of Anthony, another of the senior dancers.[14] And finally, Theresa da Costa, who plays the part of *kumadri,* is the mother of "Sub" and aunt of Beatrice, John,

Marcia, and Kelly Rodrigues (two senior and two junior dancers; an inter-
mediate sister, Ubelda, dances with Tropa de Malaca).[15] In all four cases,
these actors' formal Settlement dress—*kebaya kompridu* for the women
and suits for the men—mark them as hybridized Malaysian-Portuguese
residents of the old-time Settlement-as-housing-estate and, at the same
time, distance them from their own progeny who, in their Portuguese
costumes, represent the Settlement's mythical ancestors, the pure-blood
descendants of D'Albuquerque.

The younger-generation members of the wedding party—Sharon
Fanwell (bride), Christopher de Mello (groom), Valerie Plera (bridesmaid), and Walter Nathan (best man)—are all senior Rancho Folclorico
San Pedro dancers. For this special performance, however, they have
traded their Portuguese dance costumes for the formal clothes worn by
Settlement residents of two or three generations ago. Though they share
the same costumes as the older-generation performers, there is a crucial
difference: for Theresa and Aunty Girl, the *kebaya kompridu* they wear
are their own clothes; for Sharon and Valerie, *kebaya kompridu* are no
different from Portuguese dance wear—they are costumes worn for a
performance. Theresa and Aunty Girl may no longer wear formal dress
at contemporary Settlement weddings, but like many older Settlement
women, both continue to wear the everyday Eurasian-style *sarong kebaya*.
Young women like Sharon and Valerie, in contrast (like many other non-
Malay Malaysians), wear shorts and t-shirts on a daily basis and Western-
style dressy outfits for special occasions. For the older generation, ethnic
identity is marked in their everyday lives by dress; for the younger generation, it is marked not by dress and everyday practice but by wearing special
costumes and performing on stage.

Forging a New Synthesis

The combined cultural show and wedding scene appear superficially to
represent the two different faces of the Portuguese Settlement. Beneath
the surface, however, each half of the performance has been infiltrated by
elements from the other, leading to the forging of a new synthesis that
speaks eloquently to the ambiguities of modern Settlement life. Once
again, the musical bridges—the wedding march and the *branyo*—are crucial markers of this synthetic process. On the one hand, the wedding
march, like the myth of the direct blood link, identifies residents of the
Settlement as the descendants of D'Albuquerque. No longer part of con-

temporary Settlement life, however, the march exists solely in the sanctioned space of the cultural show. Its long-standing legitimacy, maintained primarily through ascription (it is *called* the "Portuguese wedding march"), is consolidated by its association with the costumes and music of the recently imported Portuguese half of the show. On the other hand, the *branyo,* like the suits and *kebaya kompridu* of the wedding scene, identifies residents of the Settlement as Malaysians of mixed race. The Kristang texts and melody of "Jinkly Nona" link the Settlement to a vast Portuguese diaspora that extends from Goa to Macau; the rhythm and dance steps, interchangeable with those of the *joget,* link the Settlement to long-term cultural interchange with its Malay neighbors. But the *branyo,* like the people of the Settlement, has changed its "clothes" with the times. Regardless of whether the old-time, Malay-style accompaniment of violin, *rebana,* and gong has been displaced by the "Portuguese"-style accompaniment of the cultural troupes or by the Western-style accompaniment of the current Settlement rock band, the *branyo* is still the favorite social dance of the Portuguese Settlement. In either case, its function is incorporative: different generations mix on the dance floor at Settlement weddings; different worlds mix on the stage of the Portuguese Square.

When I began this study in 1990, the Portuguese Settlement still could have been mistaken for Isabella Bird's "Sleepy Hollow." After an early morning flurry of activity during which children were roused, dressed, and packed off to school, the day settled into a leisurely routine. Before the sun got too hot, Settlement women could catch up on the latest gossip while buying fresh fish at the fishmonger's handcart or over breakfast at one of the foodstalls near the seafront. The rest of the morning was spent cooking, sweeping the house, and hand-washing clothes. The afternoon began with a half hour of noise and bustle, as hordes of uniformed girls swarmed out of the convent school towards their waiting bicycles, mopeds, and battered yellow school buses. By the time the dust settled, the Settlement was almost deserted. The only people to be seen were the old men, who enjoyed the desultory sea breeze as they alternately chatted and slept under the shady old *ketapang* tree, and a few independent tourists, who idled over cold drinks at Jenny's coffee shop (the sightseers who came in the air-conditioned tour buses rarely stopped long enough for a drink). Everyone else retreated indoors: the long, hot afternoons were for sleeping or perhaps a card game at a neighbor's house. Activity resumed once more in the late afternoon. Early evening was the most sociable time of day: bathed and powdered children spent a last few moments playing outdoors with their friends; grown-ups strolled to or from hawkers' carts, pausing briefly in front of Joe Lazaroo's house to watch the older children practice. By 10 P.M. most doors were closed to the outside world and houses were bathed in darkness, except for the telltale flickering glow of a TV set. From time to time the night calm was shattered by teenage boys racing their noisy motorbikes down D'Albuquerque Road.

The Square was almost always quiet, except for a few hours on Saturday nights, when the multicolored stage lights cast their magic and transformed it into a bustling, cosmopolitan meeting place. But when the tourists went home, the Settlement was much like any other low-income village: few cars, fewer telephones, and rickety wooden houses filled to overflowing with the children of extended families.

I have returned to the Portuguese Settlement frequently since then and have seen many changes result from the booming Malaysian economy of the early and mid-1990s. When I first arrived, for example, the primary modes of transport were motorcycles or the old green and white No. 17 town bus; today almost every household has at least one car (making parking a challenge and cycling life-threatening). Daily excursions to the open-air market are giving way to weekly expeditions by car to the supermarket at Mahkota Parade, the fancy shopping mall built on reclaimed land in Malacca Raya. The Settlement's first public payphone was installed outside No. 13 D'Albuquerque Road in late 1990; today almost every household has a telephone, many individuals have mobile phones, and a growing number of residents (including Joe Lazaroo's daughter, Elaine) are hooked up to the Internet. The Settlement even has its own web site,[1] and a new virtual diaspora is developing as residents send reports about local customs and festivals to Portuguese communities elsewhere. Real travel, too, is increasing: residents for whom Penang and Singapore seemed the ends of the earth are now flying off to visit their children in Australia, Germany, or the United States. And last, but not least, the old wooden houses with their corrugated zinc roofs and haphazard extensions are giving way one by one to stone replacements, which are less crowded because the new apartment blocks just outside the Settlement are encouraging diffusion into nuclear family homes.

● ● ●

In the midst of all this rapid social change, selected traditions provide an anchor, something comfortable and familiar that gives an illusion (at least) of stability and continuity (Hobsbawm 1983, 1–5). In order to create this illusion and at the same time foster a sense of identity and solidarity, community leaders often find themselves "involved in creatively interpreting and refashioning their customs and traditions" (Cunningham 1989,

168). In the case of the Portuguese Settlement, this creative process takes on an added dimension, for—as we have seen—the tradition for which it is best known (that of the cultural groups) is not only relatively recently invented but also was originally imported by upper-class Eurasians for a very different purpose—manufacturing a non-British European identity in the years immediately preceding independence. Like a cuckoo ejecting its hosts' natural offspring from the nest, the invented tradition has replaced older hybrid forms of music and dance, appropriating just enough of the old *branyo* to lend credibility and legitimacy to the new genre, the cultural show. The costumes, music, and dance of the cultural show form a bridge between worlds and across time. On stage, the Settlement-as-historical-monument and the Settlement-as-housing-estate, the imagined past and the experienced present, converge and forge a synthesis that is uniquely local. But what happens when the show is over? The bridge has certainly imbued the Settlement with an aura of stasis, but it is the stasis of a history that never was. As residents—especially younger-generation residents who have no memory of Clement de Silva or the first Settlement dance group—begin to believe this history, worlds begin to coalesce outside the sanctioned space of the cultural show. The cultural groups and the repertoire they perform have become absorbed into the everyday world of Settlement politics.

Anatomy of a Social Drama

Once again, by focusing on a single example, it is possible to show how this process works—how the world of the touristic borderzone and the highly political world of the Settlement-as-housing-estate intersect and interact. The case I have chosen, another episode in the increasingly complex and emotive land dispute, occurred in mid-1996. While it manifests all the elements of what Victor Turner (1986, 33–44) would call a "social drama"—a breach of the status quo, a period of doubt and discussion in which submerged divisions re-emerge as the crisis mounts, and finally some kind of resolution—it also involves three crucial elements in the residents' sense of cultural self-definition: the Settlement itself, the Festa di San Pedro, and the cultural groups. In other respects, this dispute is typical of the Settlement: the volatile tempers of leading instigators ensure that long-standing personal conflicts frequently color political posturing.

In a sense, we are coming full circle, for the subject of the dispute—the state government's ongoing land reclamation project—was introduced at the end of chapter 1.[2] Although details vary from one newspaper account to the next, by 1995, about fifteen companies had been contracted to reclaim somewhere in the region of 3,000 acres of land along a nine-mile stretch of Malacca's coastline. Two of these proposed projects will impinge directly upon Settlement life: the construction of Pulau Melaka, a resort complex built on twin man-made islands off the Bandar Hilir coast, will completely destroy the prawn breeding and spawning grounds, while the reclamation of the Settlement's seafront will physically sever the Settlement's connection to the sea, effectively relocating it a half mile inland.[3] When it became clear that development could not be stopped, the *Regedor,* his advisory panel, and the newly formed Reclamation Action Committee (RAC) began to negotiate with the state government and property developers for compensation on behalf of the Settlement community (see chapter 1).

The Breach

The longer negotiations dragged on without visible result, the more heated Settlement internal politics became. Deep distrust of the Settlement's leadership on the part of some residents combined with long-standing personal animosities on the part of others fueled the growing rift; the fact that potentially large sums of money were involved further inflamed the situation. Active fishermen, in particular, were opposed to what they perceived as the self-serving position of the leadership. From their perspective, the RAC's emphasis on preserving the integrity of the Settlement and its cultural heritage came second to securing the maximum financial reparation for loss of livelihoods. By late 1995, this increasingly vocal opposition precipitated into a new interest group, the Fishermen's Action Committee, led by a young fisherman named Gerard Danker. Tension increased as the internal breach developed external complications. On the one hand, the *Regedor's* party was firmly allied with the government (and especially with state executive councillor, Datuk Wira Gan Boon Leong); on the other, the fishermen were advised by Joseph Sta. Maria (Bernard Sta. Maria's youngest brother) and Kota Melaka MP, Lim Guan Eng, two prominent members of the opposition Democratic Action Party.[4]

Within months, two factions had developed within the Settlement: residents who were fishermen or their supporters and residents who supported the *Regedor,* his panel, and/or the RAC. This internal schism was reinforced (and complicated) by a political division between those who supported the government and those who sympathized with the opposition DAP. Although the split did not involve the entire Settlement population, those who did participate were angry, vocal, and visible. The dispute spilled into a broader forum in March, when it was announced that the 1996 Festa di San Pedro would be organized (for the second year in a row) by the *Regedor's* panel. Annual unhappiness surrounding the choice of festival organizer (a decision that invariably leads to accusations of fiscal irregularities, whomever the organizer) was magnified by the political turmoil. Despite the turmoil below the surface, an initial memorandum issued by the organizing committee provides a fascinating insight into the practice of creatively refashioning and reinterpreting local customs and "traditions":

> This feast of SAINT PETER, the Patron Saint of Fishermen and all Sea-Farers is the most celebrated and prominent traditional festival of our Malaysian Portuguese-Eurasian Community. With the observance of this age-old religious customs and the display of our rich-cultural heritage dating back to 16th. century, FESTA SAN PEDRO has now gained the status of being one of the most interesting and popular festival in MALAYSIA. This festival has attracted large crowds including local and foreign tourists resulting in its being listed as one of the attractions in the MALAYSIAN TOURIST CALENDAR. (PKKPPM 1996; emphasis in original)

The rhetoric used in this memorandum is noteworthy because it is used in the context of an internal communication from the Settlement leadership to community members, not in material addressed to outsiders.[5] It demonstrates the extent to which "the larger society's notions of tradition and cultural identity [have] become part of the rural community's self-image" (Handler and Linnekin 1984, 285). The emphases clearly pinpoint the importance of the festival to its organizers: in a nutshell, it puts the Settlement on the national map. Although there is token reference to Festa di San Pedro's religious function (as an "age-old religious custom"), more weight is placed on its status as a traditional/popular festival and tourist attraction. As the government-approved public face of the Settlement, secular cultural elements are promoted and religious aspects downplayed (see fig. 17). Mass is, indeed, celebrated, but it is held informally in the hall of the convent school rather than at the parish church of St. Peter. A priest does officiate, but it does not much matter which priest: the organizers ask whoever is willing to perform the mass and tell him when his services will be required. The priest does bless the boats, but he has

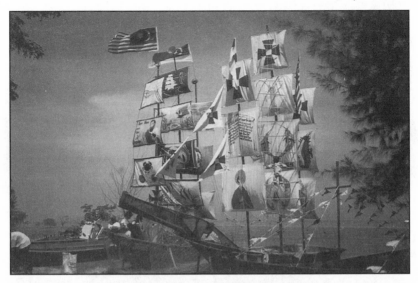

Figure 17 Preparing the boats for the decorating competition, Festa di San Pedro 1996.

become part of the spectacle—a kind of Pied Piper—a costumed actor leading the procession of residents and tourists to the sea front. In effect, he becomes a priest playing the part of a priest; he blesses boats, many of which no longer sail.[6]

The organizers also make explicit reference to the rich cultural heritage of the Settlement, which they trace back to the sixteenth century. Once again, mythical links to the world of D'Albuquerque are invoked and become crucial in imbuing the festival with an aura of authenticity. As we have seen, however, the cultural dances that feature so prominently in Festa di San Pedro entertainments do not date back to the sixteenth century. The boat decorating competition, too, is a modern invention. In fact, the festival continues to change and adapt as opportunity presents itself. For example, after the mass there is a procession from the school hall to the seafront for the blessing of the boats. Altar boys in long white robes lead the procession, waving incense and carrying crosses. They are followed by the *Irmang de Greza* (Kristang: "Brothers of the Church"), wearing their distinctive uniforms—black pants, white shirts, and short red capes—as they walk two abreast.[7] The last four *Irmang de Greza* carry a statue of Saint Peter on a palanquin full of flowers (see fig. 18). Next comes the priest (or priests, on grander occasions), who makes the sign of the cross in the general direction of each boat as he pauses to bless it. Finally, Settlement residents (carrying lighted white candles) and tourists

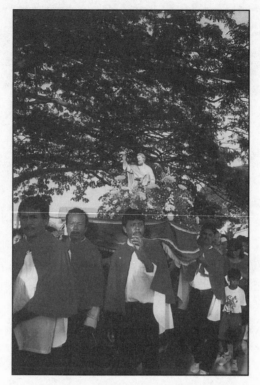

Figure 18 Irmang de Greza carrying a statue of
Saint Peter, Festa di San Pedro 1996.

form the long tail of the procession. On the surface, the whole procession
looks like a time-honored tradition. The statue of Saint Peter carried by
the *Irmang de Greza,* in particular, looks like a traditional practice that
might well be part of an Iberian-Catholic paraliturgical tradition. In fact,
this last element was introduced only in 1994, a last-minute idea derived
from other religious festivals (Good Friday, Easter Saturday, and the Feast
of the Assumption) at which statues are carried by the *Irmang de Greza.*
Although the *Irmang de Greza* attend the mass and march in the procession "out of respect to Saint Peter," participation in the procession has
not traditionally been one of their official duties (Michael Lazaroo pers.
comm., July 19, 1994). Like the priest, the *Irmang de Greza* add living
color to the overall performance.

The Crisis Mounts

The political situation deteriorated further as the Festa di San Pedro approached. Members of the fishermen's faction threatened to boycott the

boat-decorating contest (although, contrary to government attempts to secularize the festival, they still wanted to have their boats blessed by the priest) and to organize their own competing *branyo* celebration on the final evening.[8] This left the organizing committee faced with the interesting challenge of staging a fishermen's festival without the active participation of the fishermen. As the festival itself became a battleground, the two active cultural groups (Rancho Folclorico San Pedro and Tropa de Malaca) were drawn into the fray. True to form, Joe Lazaroo took the direct approach: by refusing to perform for the organizing committee, Joe appeared to ally himself with the Fishermen's Action Committee. While he may well have sympathized with the fishermen, among whom were some close friends and neighbors, Joe was more interested in withdrawing his cooperation from the *Regedor,* with whom he recently had the latest in a long series of "misunderstandings." Joe's reaction, superficially a prime example of submerged divisions re-emerging, caused near-panic for the organizers. He was not an ordinary resident: by opting out of the festival, he also withdrew his dance troupe, a crucial part of the Settlement's "rich cultural heritage dating back to sixteenth century."

With Rancho Folclorico San Pedro out of the running, Tropa de Malaca was offered all three nights of the festival. This put Noel Felix in an awkward situation. On the one hand, his younger brother was a leading member of the fishermen's faction; on the other, he had a history of cooperating with the *Regedor*—not for political reasons, but because he believed strongly in his duty to maintain the culture of the Settlement. The interdependence of the festival and its associated culture (by which he means the dance group repertoire) is clear in Noel's mind. And, as he noted, culture and politics should not mix:

> It is a tradition and it's been gazetted by the government, Margaret. It's no joke! If they gazetted in a map saying that every year we have this Festa, it's a very compulsory Festa, which the local Portuguese of Malaysians are celebrating. So now, if we don't do anything, it's going to be a mess to the community. Am I correct? I mean, forget about the *Regedor,* whatever it is, his business. But we, this is among the Festa and us and other community. Think of that. Because they are reliable on us. We have to do something for it. . . . Because why? Culture should be maintained, no matter what happen. The culture must be maintained. By hook, by crook. It must be on, because it's the identity of our races. Now, if we play politics and culture, the culture will dissolve. A politics will come up. Towards the end, nobody stand anywhere. You see. . . . So what I do, my duty is to perform

the culture only, that's all. When there's San Pedro, the culture is there. (NF, July 18, 1996)

Putting community well-being before personal preference (again, true to form), Noel decided that Tropa de Malaca should perform at the Festa di San Pedro, irrespective of the prevailing political tide. As the festival approached, however, Tropa de Malaca became a battlefield, a microcosm of the larger conflict. Parents imposed their own political agenda on their children, withdrawing them from the group if they themselves belonged to the fishermen's faction. Less than a week before the festival, the situation degenerated from social drama to soap opera. At the center of attention was Gerard Lazaroo (Tropa de Malaca's senior dancer and business manager) and his wife Merina (also a dancer). Despite having a greater measure of independence than the younger dancers (with jobs, an apartment, and two children of their own), Gerard and Merina were caught up in their parents' politics. Merina's father—Noel's brother, Patrick Felix—was so vocal in his support of the Fishermen's Action Committee that he forbade his daughter and son-in-law to perform. In contrast, Gerard's father (Emille Lazaroo) urged his son to stand up for himself and dance. In typical Settlement fashion, rumors soon abounded as observers began to "poke fire." Although the individual rumors are unimportant, the argument itself is an illuminating feature of the larger dispute, for it juxtaposes the crucial issues of filiality and "face" against the backdrop of the cultural groups and the public face of the Settlement. Gerard Lazaroo was faced with a difficult choice: to respect his father-in-law, who insisted that he would lose face if Gerard danced; to be the filial son and follow his own father's advice (and allow his father-in-law to lose face); or to lose face himself by letting the group down and allowing himself, an adult with children of his own, to be publicly treated like a child by his father-in-law.

The Resolution

The solution for Gerard was a relatively straightforward pragmatic compromise. He did not put on his costume, nor did he dance; instead, he attended the performances in everyday clothes and stood at the back of the stage as manager and chief cheerleader. Noel Felix's dilemma was far more complex: he had agreed to perform for the sake of the community but no longer had enough experienced dancers available. With only a week to go before the opening night, Noel was faced with the challenge of trying to train a new group of dancers from scratch. To avoid inflaming the political situation further, Noel moved practices from Tropa de Mala-ca's usual semipublic space (the back yard of the kindergarten school near the Square) to the front yard of Josephine and Domingos de Costa's house on the periphery of the Settlement (at A1 Eredia Road—see map 2), well away from prying eyes. Noel's task was enormous: none of the regular musicians were available to play for afternoon practices, only one of the new dancers had any previous experience (with the disbanded D'Tiru-Tiru group), and one of his (unavailable) regular dancers objected strongly to the newcomers being allowed to join Tropa de Malaca on a permanent basis.

By the time the festival began, however, Noel had transformed what promised to be a major disaster into three successful performances. With too little time to train a full complement of new dancers, he arrived at an inspired solution to his predicament: he staged a short informal wedding scene followed by an abbreviated cultural dance show. In practical terms, the wedding scene occupied the stage, making a cultural show given by a minimum complement of three couples feasible and giving the trainee dancers (who deserved some kind of reward for their efforts) a less stressful stage debut as members of the wedding scene cast. At the same time, Noel's strategy appeared to suggest that the cultural dance tradition claimed by the Settlement as its own (linking residents back to the sixteenth century) was not naturally coursing through the veins of its youth and that the wedding scene was, in fact, more representative of its indigenous, racially mixed Eurasian heritage. Furthermore, when the dancers in their Portuguese costumes entertained the mixed-race Eurasians of the wedding scene, the ambiguity of the Settlement's present appeared in sharp relief. While Portuguese dance may not be indigenous, it has become a living part of the lives of the dancers: it is their tradition.

On the first night, Noel started out with a skeleton crew: three regular members of Tropa de Malaca (two girls and one boy), one former dancer (a girl), one new dancer (a boy who had been a leading dancer with D'Tiru-Tiru before the group was disbanded), and Anne de Mello (Gerard de Costa's wife), who was persuaded to come out of "retirement" and to make up numbers by dancing as a boy. But the Festa di San Pedro is the traditional time when everyone—including young men who have left Malacca in search of work—comes home to celebrate. By the third night, three old boys who had returned from Singapore and Kuala Lumpur for the festival had relieved Anne of the need to cross-dress. Ignoring Settlement politics, the former dancers put on their costumes and joined their friends on stage. It was clear from the joy on their faces, their sheer delight in the act of dancing, and all the old jokes flying around the stage that the tradition they were performing for the entertainment of the wedding scene cast and tourists alike was their own.

Closing Thoughts

As I have suggested throughout this book, the Portuguese Settlement is not a modern-day Sleepy Hollow full of Rip van Winkles magically transported from the sixteenth century. Instead, two Settlements coexist in time and space. One is a community no different from any other rapidly developing low-income community. The other Settlement, which exists in the pages of guidebooks and in the imaginations of tourists, is filled with ghosts from the past and reflects the ephemeral experience of tourists themselves. Residents pass between the worlds with consummate ease: they come home from work, put on their costumes, pick up their guitars, and head towards the stage, for the stage is the meeting ground. Music and dance constitute their public face; all else remains invisible. When the lights in the Square begin to dim and the music begins, myth, illusion, and reality gently collide and coalesce.

The imaginary Settlement temporarily transcends reality to become the romantic, authentic, timeless place tourists want to find. The transformation is not necessarily as innocent as it might appear, for it also provides a powerful means of promoting particular ways of seeing (and of not seeing) the world. In effect, the Settlement becomes a forum within which diverse messages can compete and speak simultaneously to different audiences. It constitutes a potential opportunity that the government—adept at manipulating all kinds of symbols in the process of nation building—has been quick to exploit. Viewed in this light, the government's construction of the Portuguese Square represents a clear attempt to convert the Settlement from a rather unusual housing estate into a historical monument. By promoting the Settlement under the guise of tourism, the government covertly coopts it for political and economic gain.

The package, however, works differently for different audiences; each tourist constructs a past that is individually meaningful (Bruner 1994, 410). Western tourists are presented with what superficially appears to be a Malaysian version of Colonial Williamsburg. But the fact remains that it is a replica of a history that never was. Women do not stroll around the Settlement wearing the rustic Portuguese folk costumes one sees on stage. Instead, old women wear the same Malay-style *sarong kebaya*s their grandmothers wore before them, and young girls wear shorts and T-shirts. Domestic (Malaysian and Singaporean) and regional (primarily Japanese and Korean) audiences, in contrast, see a very different picture: Settlement residents, seemingly displayed in their natural habitat, become exoticized objects, vestiges of a colonial era that has been tamed and contained in a theme park. As we displayed Asian people in re-created "authentic" environments at our World's Fairs, so now the Malaysian government symbolically displays its power over make-believe Europeans. That the "Europeans" are represented as Portuguese—the most distant of all colonial intruders—and not as Dutch or British is hardly surprising. The romantic aura, stereotypical easygoing nature, and low social status of the Portuguese community are less threatening to the government today than references to more oppressive recent colonial regimes.

Having demonstrated their power over these vestigial "Europeans," the government uses the cultural show to send a broader message. Sanctioned nationwide as a legitimate showcase for "traditional" performing arts, the cultural show has become one of the few venues at which overt manifestations of non-Malay ethnic identity is actively encouraged (albeit reduced to three-minute "soundbites"). Such performances, aimed at local as well as international audiences, reinforce the illusion of happy multicultural coexistence in a setting that poses no threat to the fragile status quo. This illusion, however, disguises the growing segregation in the arts. Just as *bangsawan* and *zapin* were transformed from popular cosmopolitan genres into "traditional Malay performing arts" so, too, has the performing tradition of the Portuguese Settlement been transformed from hybrid Malaysian-Portuguese genres *(branyo* and *mata kantiga)* into an ethnically distinct "Portuguese" genre (the cultural show).

But what of the people of the Settlement? By grasping their opportunities they have navigated the ups and downs of post-independence Malaysia more successfully than any other minority. In the late 1960s, wearing *sarongs* and *kebayas*, dancing to the beat of the *branyo,* and song duelling, they demonstrated their status as long-standing members of the Malaysian family. The resemblance of *joget* and *dondang sayang* to *branyo* and *mata kantiga* suggests long-term musical interaction between the two communities, an interaction culminating in the widespread acceptance of "Jinkly Nona" as national property. That Portuguese influence on Malay traditional music is universally accepted—but never defined, except in the vaguest terms—further reinforces their deep interconnectedness. Trying to pin down exactly what constitutes "Portuguese influence" in Indonesia, Tilman Seebass (n.d., 29–30) reaches the same impasse, finally reiterating the generally held opinion: Portuguese influence is there, but it is so deep-seated that it is no longer possible to isolate particular characteristics.

Portuguese music and dance has become such an integral part of Settlement life that the *Regedor* frequently exhorts young dancers to "keep up their culture." Ironically, by becoming less Malaysian and more "ethnic," Settlement residents can now take advantage of benefits such as savings bonds schemes otherwise open only to ethnic Malays.[9] Yet, while undoubtedly not Malaysian, the repertoire of the cultural groups can no longer be considered completely Portuguese. Over the years, it has become something distinctly Kristang: texts no longer make sense in modern Portuguese, new songs have been composed in the same style, and dance movements have become smoother and more gracefully Malay. After a half century the tradition is no longer invented and the community no longer imagined.

Despite the widespread fame and recognition accorded to Settlement performing troupes, it is increasingly apparent that there are strings attached. The Settlement owes its position to the central role it occupies in the government-created "Historical Malacca" package: success is only tolerated within these confines.[10] Although residents are encouraged and rewarded for excellence in the cultural sphere—the forum deemed acceptable by the government—they are discriminated against in other musical domains. In late 1992, for example, Joe Lazaroo and Rancho Folclorico San Pedro were voted "the best cultural troupe in the state during the recent Malacca Tourism Week celebrations" (*The Star,* November 2, 1992). A few weeks earlier, however, Basil Bournaparte (Joe's drummer) and his pop music band, The Vintage, were the subjects of a lengthy national newspaper feature exposing the way leading Kuala Lumpur hotels discriminate against local bands in general and Malaysian-Portuguese bands in particular. The Vintage, described as "a popular group from the Portuguese Settlement in Malacca," had their contract with the Pan-Pacific Hotel terminated to make way for a four-piece Indonesian group (*NST,* September 26, 1992).[11] When it comes to strolling around a five-star hotel singing American and Malay popular songs, Malacca-Portuguese musicians—no matter how good they might be—are no longer "exotic" enough.

In the final analysis, there is a sense in which the story of this remarkable community and its history come into conflict. In other words, this book has two quite different endings. One is happy; the other has yet to be written. One is descriptive history; the other is prescriptive story.[12] The first ending suggests that residents have seized their opportunities and managed both to translate negative ethnic stereotypes (lazy, music-loving Portuguese-Eurasians) into positive role models (glamorous, hard-working keepers of culture) and to carve a new niche for themselves within the Malaysian nation. None of the developments—the creation of the Settlement, the introduction and eclectic accumulation of Portuguese music and dance, or even the recent tourist boom—were of their own initiation, but pragmatic adaptability has been the key to their success as residents have gone on to improvise a culture purely their own. When Joe Lazaroo comments that "dancing is a part of the Portuguese way of life and many are good dancers. . . . [Though we] dance to celebrate festivals and to add cheer, nowadays we also dance for tourists" (*MM,* September 26, 1992), he shares an important truth but omits to make clear that the dances performed for Settlement celebrations and those performed for tourists are not the same.

The second ending has yet to be written. On the one hand, it seems as though the Settlement, in its most creative phase of performing self, is slipping away. As scholars we can lament the passing of old-time *mata kantiga* and *branyo.* The new Portuguese dance tradition, too, is in a transitional phase as major performers and organizers are passing away or retiring and younger-generation performers are still finding their feet. On the other hand, the vital signs are good and hold out hope for the future. The *branyo,* in its modern rock-band manifestation, is still the most popular social dance at Settlement celebrations and continues to unite the generations on the dance floor. Young musicians and dancers, who have grown up with Portuguese dance all around them, no longer feel obliged to repeat what Clement de Silva or any of the Upper Tens taught their parents and grandparents. Having internalized a repertoire of music and movement, they are consciously starting to create something purely their own. The history of the Settlement and its people has always been one of constant adaptation and flexibility. Though the world is considerably smaller and the threats to the integrity of their land loom much larger, I see no reason for that to change. Ever the optimist, I look forward to seeing what happens when my godson Jeremy is old enough to join the dance.

Musical Examples

The transcriptions and lyrics included here are for the three pieces discussed in chapter four and the items included in the cultural show described in chapter five. Of course, this represents a small sample of the total repertoire of the cultural dance groups. The lyrics of a broader selection of songs and dances can be found in the booklet accompanying the CD *Kantiga di Padri sǎ Chang* (Sarkissian 1998).

Texts originally set in Kristang (e.g., "Jinkly Nona," "Vira di Bairu Portuguès," and "Vira Sta. Marta") are easily transcribed and translated into English. Texts originally set in Portuguese, however, present more complex challenges for the transcriber/translator (as is demonstrated in chap. 4).

Because these songs have been transmitted orally, singers often approximate sounds or even substitute Kristang words or phrases. In most of these cases, I have tried to transcribe the words exactly as they are sung (following Baxter's orthography for Kristang, where possible), but because coherent translation is often impossible, I have generally used Portuguese versions for English translation. I am grateful to the Portuguese ethnomusicologist Susana Sardo for her invaluable assistance in tracking down Portuguese originals, and to my colleagues Charles Cutler and David Jackson for assistance with the texts for "Ti' Anika," "Camacha," and "Baile de Roda." In the case of "Camacha" and "Regadinyo," which are performed as instrumental numbers by everyone except Joe Lazaroo, Portuguese versions of the texts from Joe's files are given (hence the Portuguese spelling of *regadinho*, a word of which Sardo notes, "It's so usual to sing this song all around the country [i.e., Portugal], that our language already absorbs the word *regadinho*. We know the word, we know that it is related with water, but we don't know what it means" (pers. comm., Jan. 9, 2000). The text to "Baile de Roda" remains problematic: the version that appears in Lazaroo's collection was typed by someone who did not know Portuguese. The second verse has been identified by Susana Sardo as a common Portuguese text; the first verse, however, is unclear.

Example 1　Mma-să filu

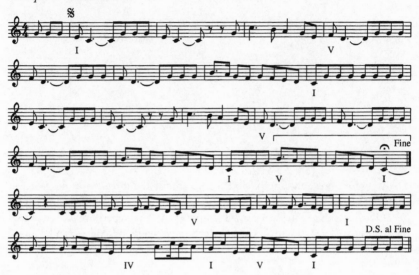

Mama-să filu	Mummy's boy
Mama-să filu	Mummy's boy
Keré chupá su chupeta	Wants to suck his dummy
Undi teng chupeta	Where's the dummy
Undi teng chupeta	Where's the dummy
Trazé chupeta	Bring the dummy
Baté peu kong song *churá*	Stamp feet, [no meaning] cry
Mama-să filu	Mummy's boy
Mama-să filu	Mummy's boy
Keré chupá su chupeta	Wants to suck his dummy
Undi teng chupeta	Where's the dummy
Undi teng chupeta	Where's the dummy
Tomá chupeta	Take the dummy
Bai chupá kera-kera	Go suck, [don't get cross]
Filu păkăninu	Little boy
Mama-să korasang	Mummy's heart
Bai lá nă mufinu	Go away, devil
Beng bong *nă si churang*	[Be nice?] to the cry baby
Undi teng chupeta	Where's the dummy
Ke peta *tă churá*	The little one's crying
Kara *di chupeta*	Dummy face
Bai chupá kera-kera	Go suck, [don't get cross]

Example 2 Ti' Anika

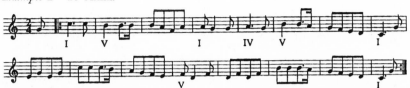

| *Joe Lazaroo* | | *Noel Felix* |
| (typed, n.d.) | | (oral, 1990) |

Olé, olá	*Olé, olá*	*Olé, olá*
Esta vida não está má	This life's not so bad	*Engsabida nus toma*
Olá, olé	*Olá, olé*	*Olá, olé*
Ti Anica de Loulae	Aunty Annie from Loulé	*Ti' Anika di lolay*
Ti' Anica, Anica	Aunty Annie, Annie	*Ti' Anika, Anika*
Ti' Anica de Fuzeta	Aunty Annie from Fuseta	*Ti' Anika ja fuzayta*
A quem desejaria ela	I wonder to whom she gave	*Agienda ira ela*
Asaia da bara preta	The skirt with the black border	*Azianda bara preta*
Olé, olá, etc.	*Olé, olá*, etc.	*Olé, olá*, etc.
Asaia da bara preta	The skirt with the black border	*Azianda bara preta*
A bara do cachine	The edging of ?	*Abaranda kashiné*
Ti' Anica, mana'nica	Aunty Annie, sister Annie	*Ti' Anika manda'nika*
Ti' Anica de Loulae	Aunty Annie from Loulé	*Ti Anika di lolay*
Olé, olá, etc.	*Olé, olá*, etc.	*Olé, olá*, etc.

Example 3 Jinkly Nona

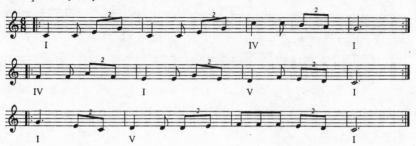

Malacca, 1964
(Knowlton 1964)

Jingli nonă jingli nonă	Sinhalese girl, Sinhalese girl	*Jinkly Nona, Jinkly Nona*
Yo kerê kazá	I want to marry (you)	*Yo keré kazá*
Kază num tem portă	(Your) house has no door	*Kaza nunteng potra, Nona*
Ki laia logu pasá?	How (am I) to enter?	*Kái logu pasá?*

Malacca, 1991

Sri Lanka, 1894
(Fernando 1894)

Cingalee Nona! Cingalee Nona!	Sinhalese girl, Sinhalese girl!
Eu kere kasa	I want to marry you
Porta ninkere, orta ninkere	I do not want your house or garden
Figa namas da	Just give (me) your daughter

Example 4 Fara Pera

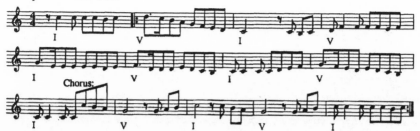

Leça
(published, ca. 1983)

Chamaste-me farrapeira	Call me *farrapeira*
Eu nunca vendi farrapos	I never sold old clothes
Tenho uma camisa nova	I have a new shirt
Toda cheia de buracos	That's all full of holes

Joe Lazaroo
(oral, 1990)

[chorus]
A e o lay (× 4)

Chamastema fara pera
Yo nungka vendi perapus
A e o lay
Yo nungka vendi perapus
Teng ungwa saia nova
Toda chea di burakos
Chamastema fara pera
Yo nungka vendi perapus

[chorus]
A e o lay (× 4)

Gerard de Costa
(oral, 1991)

[chorus]
A e o lay (× 4)

O minya fara peresta
O minya fara perona
A e o lay
Fara pera
[unclear]
[unclear] *alegra*
O minya pera
Nus tă kantá tă balá

[chorus]
A e o lay (× 4)

Example 5   Ao Nosso Algarve

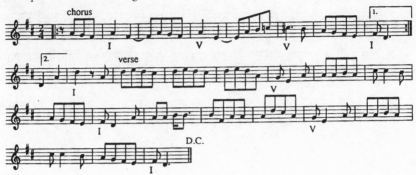

Chorus

Ao nos' Algarve	To our Algarve
De seu azul	With the blue sky
Kantai kantiga	Sing songs
Linda figueré de sul	Beautiful fig trees of the south
O m' linda algarvia	Oh my beautiful Algarvian girl
Kuma tu na ha igual	There's no one like you
E mossa sa bonita	You're the most beautiful girl
Teras de Portugal	In the lands of Portugal
Para mim es um santa	To me you are a saint
O raīnya da aldeia	Oh queen of the village
Para mim es' semente	To me you are the seed
Káida ke Deus semeya	Sown by God
Ao nos' Algarve, etc.	To our Algarve, etc.

Example 6   Vira di Sta. Marta

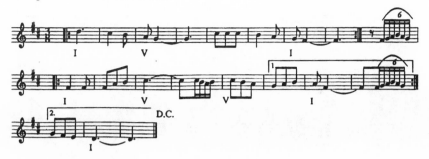

Beng nus bai kantá	Come, let's sing
Ki fazé tudu nus santá	Why are we sitting
Beng nus bai bailá	Come, let's dance
Vira di Santa Marta	The *vira* from Santa Marta
Vira Santa Marta	*Vira* Santa Marta
Nus bailá	We dance
Para jenti fazé alegria	To make people happy
Vira Santa Marta	*Vira* Santa Marta
Nus bailá	We dance
Isti festa fazé nossa dia	This festival makes our day
Beng kantá	Come sing
Beng bailá	Come dance
Vira di Santa Marta, olé	*Vira* from Santa Marta, *olé*

Example 7   O Malhão (Joe's version)

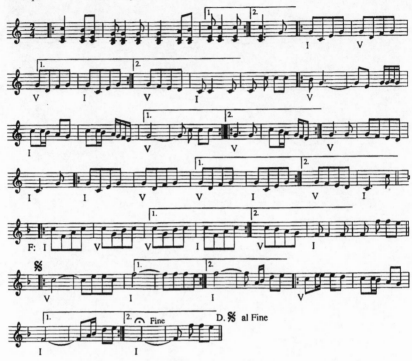

[instrumental introduction]

O malhão tris' malhão	Oh *malhão,* sad *malhão*
O malhão tris' malhão	Oh *malhão,* sad *malhão*
Ai o vinyu	Ai, the wine
O malhão tris' koitadu	Oh *malhão,* poor sad one
Uma, dos, trés e vira	One, two, three, and turn
Uma, dos, trés e vira	One, two, three, and turn
Ai o vinyu	Ai, the wine
Vira ke dansa o malhão	Long live the one who dances the *malhão*

[instrumental interlude]

O malhão, malhão	Oh *malhão, malhão*
Ki vidé a tua	What a life for you
Ko moré vivé	Eating and drinking
O ti rim tim tim	Oh, *terrim-tim-tim*
Pasiyá nau rua	Strolling in the street

Example 7 (continued)

O malhão, malhão	Oh *malhão, malhão*
O malhão aki	Oh *malhão* here
Si dansa dansi	If you dance, dance
O ti rim tim tim	Oh, *terrim-tim-tim*
Sa fugé fugé	If you flee, flee

Example 8 Camacha

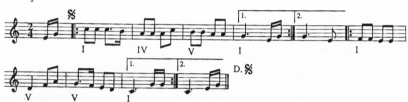

Dei-te dois beijos Maria	I gave you two kisses, Maria
Tu deste-os muito depois	You gave them back much later
Sabes que a casa não queria	You know that my family didn't agree
Portanto dá cá mais dois.	So, give me two more.
Se fossemos para o coreto	If we went to the bandstand
Teu pai não consentiria	Your father would not allow it
Mas esta noite em segredo	But tonight, in secret
Dei-te dois beijos Maria	I gave you two kisses, Maria.

Example 9   Regadinho

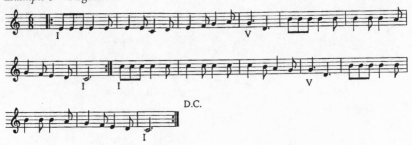

Água leva o regadinho	The *regadinho* carries water
Água leva o regador	The watering can carries water
Enquanto rega e não rega	While it is and isn't watering
Vira-te para mim amor.	Turn to me, my love

Example 10   Tiru Liru Liru

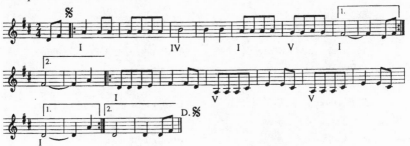

La em śima sta o tiru liru liru	Up there, there's *tiru-liru-liru*
Ka em baśu sta o tiru liru lo	Down there, there's *tiru-liru-lo*
Juntadu-se os dois ar esquinas	They meet each other on the corner
A tocado konsertina	Playing the concertina
A dansá o solidó	Dancing the *solidó*
Kumadri minya kumadri	Godmother, my godmother
Yo gosto da sua pakena	I like your little one
E bonito prazantá sa beng	She's beautiful, she's well presented
Paresa ke teng, a fasa morena	It seems that she's dark skinned

Example 11   Baile de Roda

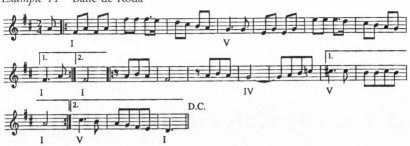

Isti bailarico novo	This new *bailarico*
Que esta vi daqui este picado	That has come here for this show
Eles su dos rapados	Two boys
Sentá perto pé furado	Are seated nearby with ready feet

A moda do bailarico	The *moda* [style] of *bailarico*
Não tem nada que saber	Isn't difficult to dance
É bailar com um pé no ar	We dance with one foot in the air
Outro no chão a bater.	And the other stamping on the floor.

[Chorus, in Kristang, × 2]

A e o lay	*A e o lay*
A e o lay	*A e o lay*
Beng nus baila balinyu Portuguès	Let's dance the Portuguese dance

Example 12 Vira di Bairu Português

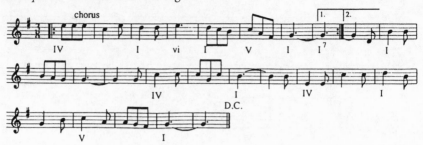

Chorus

Beng nus kantá, beng nus bailá	Come let's sing, come let's dance
Vira di bairu Português	The *vira* of the Portuguese Settlement
Ja fiká nã bairu Português	In the Portuguese Settlement
Sã jenti gostá alegrá	Its people like to enjoy themselves
Beng San Juang, San Pedro	[When the feasts of] St. John and St. Peter come
Tudu lembrá, fazé isti dia alegria	Everyone remembers and makes the day happy

[chorus]   [chorus]

Jenti di bairu Português	The people of the Portuguese Settlement
Trabaliá nã tera ku mar	Work on land and at sea
Gadrá dinyiru per isti úngua dia	They save their money for this one day
Alegrá ku mulé familia	And are happy with their wives and families

[chorus]   [chorus]

Jenti di bairu Português	The people of the Portuguese Settlement
De sperá dia di Natal	Wait for Christmas Day
Tisé sibrisu per isti úngua dia	They mend their clothes for this one day
Alegrá fazé alegria	And are happy enjoying themselves

[chorus]

Notes

Introduction

1.   For all the accordionists out there, I played Joe Lazaroo's ancient Baile accordion. This Chinese-made instrument had 32 bass buttons, a piano keyboard with a range of a little over two octaves, and no additional voices. While this basic instrument was fine for playing Portuguese dance music, it was not suitable for playing in the more melodically melismatic Malay style. Malay accordionists prefer the extended keyboard of the 120-bass instrument, although they never use any of the bass buttons.

2.   A political cartoon that appeared in the March 10, 1991 issue of the *New Straits Times* captures this image perfectly. Drawn by Lat, Malaysia's most famous cartoonist, the cartoon depicts the Malaysian general public's view of the Portuguese Settlement. Members of the proposed Portuguese Settlement branch of UMNO (United Malays National Organization, the dominant party in the ruling coalition government)—depicted as musicians and dancers in Portuguese dress with guitars raised, ready to perform at the drop of a hat—stand in line beside branch members from adjacent Malay villages, all motionless and wearing Islamic dress.

3.   The notion of coexisting/competing histories, which I have called "history as imagined" and "history that actually happened," grew naturally out of my data and my knowledge of the Portuguese Settlement. As so often happens when one has good ideas that seem to make sense, I later discovered that Edward Shils (1981, 195) made the same point far more eloquently: "There are two pasts. One is the sequence of occurred events, of actions which were performed and of the actions which they called forth, moving through a complex sequence of actions until the present is reached. . . . There is another past. This is the perceived past. This is a much more plastic thing, more capable of being retrospectively reformed by human beings living in the present. It is the past which is recorded in memory and in writing, formed from encounters with 'the hard facts,' not just from inescapable but also from sought-for encounters."

4. Mousedeer (*kancil* in Malay) is the colloquial term for a chevrotain, a small deer-like animal *(Tragulus pygmaeus)*. This particular mousedeer, known by the proper name Sri Kancil, has become both an emblem for the state of Malacca and a Malaysian folk "hero" (in which capacity "he" is probably more famous than Parameswara himself). There are countless children's stories about the clever mousedeer who outwits larger, stronger animals.

5. According to recent statistics, about 57 percent of Malaysia's 18 million inhabitants are ethnically "Malay." Of the remainder, 32 percent are categorized as "Chinese," 9 percent as "Indian," and 2 percent as "Other" (Central Intelligence Agency 1994). The fact that such statistics exist suggests, as Joel Kahn (1992, 62) has pointed out, that racial definitions of this sort are straightforward and unproblematic. But the statistics disguise deeper complexities. For example, it is far from clear what being *Malay* actually means. As Clive Kessler (1992, 139–40) demonstrates, the standard definition of a "Malay"—one who is *bumiputra* (indigenous, lit.: "son of the soil") and Islamic—does not account adequately for Malay *bumiputra* who are not Muslim (e.g., certain aboriginal groups), for *bumiputra* Muslims who are not Malay (e.g., the Melanau of Sarawak), or for Muslim Malays who are not *bumiputra* (e.g., Acehnese immigrants from Sumatra). Further, it does not account for Malays who are neither *bumiputra* nor Muslim (e.g., Javanese and Batak Christian immigrants), for *bumiputra* who are neither Muslim nor Malay (e.g., ethnic Thai Buddhists and some tribal populations in East Malaysia), nor for Muslims who are neither Malay nor *bumiputra* (e.g., Indians, Arabs, etc.).

The labels "Chinese" and "Indian" mask equally broad categories, encompassing people who speak distinct dialects or languages, profess diverse religions, who came to Malaysia for different reasons at divergent points in history from disparate parts of their home subcontinents. Within these broader categories "Chinese" and "Indian" are two distinct subgroups, centered in Malacca and known locally as the Baba-Nonya (*Peranakan* or Straits-born Chinese) and Chitty Melaka (*Chittys* or Straits-born Indian) communities. Descended from early traders who settled in Malacca (and may or may not have married locally), both communities have resided in Malaysia for so long that their language, dress, food, and many other customs—except religion—are effectively Malay. Members of these hybridized communities consider themselves distinct from the majority of immigrants from China and India, who began to arrive during British times. The term "Straits-born" seems to have originated during the early days of the British Straits Settlements, a time when there would have been a distinction between the older, established trading communities and the newly arrived Chinese and Indians. The Malacca Baba-Nonya community has been extensively studied by Tan Chee Beng (1988).

The fact that the Baba-Nonya and Chitty Melaka communities are of longer standing than some more recent Islamic immigrants makes the criteria for *bumiputra* status seem arbitrary. And this does not even begin to consider communities lumped together under the label "Other." The *orang asli* (aboriginal peoples) and Portuguese Eurasians (some of whom trace their residency back four centuries), to give just two examples, are considered *bumiputra* for some purposes but not for others, yet neither are considered "Malay" (Kessler 1992, 139–40). For a similar discussion of anomalous population elements with specific reference to Malacca, see Clammer 1986, 54–60.

6. See, for example, Rubenstein 1992.

7. In contrast to the limited number of professional troupes (supported by the national government and by individual state governments), there are literally dozens of small amateur or semi-professional cultural troupes all over Malaysia. They perform not only for tourists but also in response to a growing urban domestic market. Cultural shows are now in big demand, whether it be in conjunction with local festivals or food promotions at fancy hotels, as floorshows for company dinners, or even (most recently) as entertainment to enliven rapidly proliferating shopping malls. Though they vary greatly in ability and longevity, these troupes have one thing in common: organization along ethnic lines. Encouraged by a government eager to send messages of multicultural diversity and harmonious coexistence to internal and external audiences, grassroots cultural troupes take advantage of this opportunity to express ethnic difference publicly. Frequently performing alongside cultural troupes from other ethnic groups, they visually demonstrate multicultural diversity. Harmonious coexistence, however, is another matter. Performers from different cultural troupes may share a stage, but they often remain ethnically segregated, even behind the scenes. To give a practical example, during a year of performing at Saturday night cultural shows at the Portuguese Square, where there were at least three ethnically distinct cultural troupes present on any single occasion, I never witnessed any interaction between performers of different ethnic backgrounds. Youngsters who shared a changing room on a regular basis barely acknowledged each other. Even negotiations about the performing order for the evening were directed through an emcee supplied by the State Economic Development Corporation. As soon as the SEDC ceded the running of the Square to the Portuguese Settlement Development Board, the multicultural shows stopped; today one can only see Portuguese troupes performing at the Square on a Saturday night.

Chapter One

1. Texeira's source is Francisco de Souza's two-volume *O Oriente conquistado a Jesus Christo pelos Padres da Companhia de Jesus* (Lisbon, 1710), pt. 1, 225.

2. No daily newspapers were published in Malacca. Local papers issued on a weekly or fortnightly basis were mostly short lived: the *Malacca Guardian*

(2 January 1928 to 30 December 1940), the *Malacca Observer* (3 November 1924 to 26 December 1927), and *Suara Benar* (September 1932 to February 1933). All are available on microfilm at the British Library Newspaper Division.

3. Today only a handful of Eurasian families remain in Tranquerah (Tengkera in Malay). The wealthiest emigrated after Malaysian independence. Of those who stayed, some moved to the new suburbs of Bukit Baru and Bukit Beruang; others, in more modest circumstances, built homes in the Portuguese Settlement, not far from the old Praya Lane *kampung*.

4. The full text of the speech is given below, followed by my own translation. Judging from the syntax, which is neither distinctly Portuguese nor reflective of Malay word order (more common in modern Kristang), it appears as though the text was translated from English into Kristang.

> Nos descendente de Portuguez que sta fica na este terra de Malacca pertence a Egreja de missao Portuguez juntar hoji naqui para presentar nossa grande respeito com Excellentissimo Senhor como ungha representador de Governmente de Portugal na este primeiro visita de Excellentissimo Senhor na Malacca.
>
> Nos toma esta occasion para fala com senhor que nos tan tanto alegria para encontra com senhor que nos tem contenti para dar saber com senhor que nos senti muito gabado que nos ja desce de filho de Portugal que com sua valenti accao ja faze com eloutro premeiro descobridor de Oriente. Nos lembra que Excellentissimo senhor tamem tan tanto alegria por saber que ainda quatro cento anno ja passa desnao Don Albuquerque ja Macar este terra, nos sta linguage Portuguez e segni costume de Portuguez.
>
> Nos pedi com senhor para recebe nossa grande merce porque senhor a toma tanto trabalho por visita nossa pobre terra.
>
> Adeus senhor e senhora e familia.
>
> Nos vos humilde serbidor. (*MG*, April 22, 1929)

We Portuguese descendants, who live in this land of Malacca and belong to the church of the Portuguese Mission, gather here today to pay our respects to you, illustrious Senhor, as a representative of the Portuguese government on [the occasion of] your first visit to Malacca.

We take this opportunity to inform you that we are most happy to meet you and are honored to descend from the son of Portugal who, through his brave deeds, was the first discoverer of the Orient. With great joy we remind you that even though four hundred years have passed since Don Albuquerque arrived in this land, we still speak the language and follow the customs of Portugal.

We ask you to receive our sincerest thanks for taking the trouble to visit our poor land.

Goodbye to you, Senhor, and to your wife and family.

Your humble servants.

5. No one is sure what "Upper Tens" meant originally; some residents suggest it might refer to the upper ten percent of the community. The term is still used today by members of the Portuguese Settlement to describe someone who is (or thinks he is) of a higher social class.

6. The list of wedding presents alone covered two columns of small print (*MG*, January 20, 1936). Ida de Silva (née Rodrigues), born in 1914, remained an active pianist throughout her life. Her husband, Clement de Silva, held the post of choirmaster at St. Peter's Church for over thirty-five years. After Clement's death in 1969, Ida moved to Kuala Lumpur, ending her involvement with musical life in Malacca. In 1976 she emigrated to Australia and became involved as pianist with a dance group established in 1990 by the rapidly growing Perth Malacca Portuguese community. Ida passed away in late 1997.

7. The first Eurasian Company, established in 1902 as a branch of the Singapore Volunteer Corps, was disbanded in 1906 after the commanding officer, Resident Councillor R. N. Bland, was transferred from Malacca. A. J. Minjoot, secretary of the rural board and Member of the British Empire (M.B.E.), had served in 1902 with the original Eurasian company. Captain of the Volunteers until 1933, Minjoot finally transferred to the Reserve Officers due to indifferent health; he was succeeded by Captain E. V. Rodrigues, another leading socialite and father of the Sports Club's Ida (Eurasian Association, Penang 1934a, 22).

8. Novelty items of this sort were introduced via 78 rpm recordings. Tan Sooi Beng notes that about 0.6 million gramophone records were imported to Malaya in 1929 from the United Kingdom, the United States, and Germany. While the earliest recordings were almost certainly bought by resident expatriates, by the 1920s the rapidly growing urban population constituted a large domestic market (Tan Sooi Beng 1996–97, 6–7).

9. Perhaps predictably, the Singapore and Penang communities were first to organize. The Singapore Recreation Club (established in 1883) and the Eurasian Literary Association (founded in 1918) merged in 1919 to become the Singapore Eurasian Association (Eurasian Association, Singapore 1989, 24). The latter was already active when Penang Eurasians founded an organization on November 1, 1919 (A.M.F. 1935, 14; Eurasian Association, Penang 1987, i), followed closely by Selangor on December 14. Initial enthusiasm soon faded: the associations continued, but their activities were minimal until a revival occurred in the mid-1930s. In 1934, for example, the Selangor Eurasian Association was "practically dormant, but a new interest was awakened" among the younger generation (Eurasian Association, Penang 1934b, 12). This new interest spread nationwide: Negri Sembilan had an active association by October 1934 and Perak was in the process of organizing before the idea was even mooted in Malacca, despite the fact that Malacca had by far the largest concentration of Eurasians in the country (H. M. de Souza, quoted in Howell 1934, 23). Kedah, the last state

to organize, formed its Eurasian Association between September and December 1936.

10. The committee included H. M. de Souza, J.P. (President), D. Theseira (Vice President), E. W. Howell (Secretary), C. F. Gomes (Treasurer), R. S. de Souza, A. J. Minjoot, M.B.E., and Capt. E. V. Rodrigues. Once again, we can see the tightly knit structure of Upper Tens society. Many of the committee members also served the community in other contexts. For example, D. Theseira and R. S. de Souza (speech-maker for the governor of Macau's visit in 1929) were both on the board of the newly formed Portuguese Settlement Committee; H. M. de Souza, J.P., was Chairman of the Malacca Girls' Sports Club; and E. V. Rodrigues and A. J. Minjoot, M.B.E., led the Eurasian Volunteers.

11. The same negative stereotypes continue to haunt Settlement residents to the present and, as we shall see below, are only now being countered in some small measure by their national prominence achieved through music and dance.

12. Community activists believe that the twenty-five original lots had Dutch titles and freehold status; the amalgamated lot, which covered 28.125 acres and was given a new number (Lot 248), apparently retained its freehold status (B. Sta. Maria 1982, 128; J. Sta. Maria 1994, 8). The official survey department file, SDM 393/31 (Survey Department, Malacca, file number 393 of 1931), reproduced in B. Sta. Maria 1982, 129, refers to an earlier file, LOM 453/27 (Land Office, Malacca, file number 453 of 1927). This earlier file is believed to "contain details of status and ownership of the settlement land . . . [and] a copy of the land grant given to the church stating that it is freehold land" (*Sunday Star,* October 25, 1987). Unfortunately, LOM 453/27 is "missing." In the absence of proof, successive British and Malaysian governments have repossessed portions of land, revoked the freehold status, and issued first Temporary Occupation Licenses (TOL) and later ninety-nine- and sixty-year leases.

13. The first four committee members were J. R. Neave, Fr. J. P. François, Fr. A. M. Coroado, and Captain Percy, respectively. Theseira, the honorary secretary, and de Souza were both upper-class Eurasians who later also served on the Malacca Eurasian Association committee. As for the priests, it was apparently "most remarkable to see these two missionaries, one from the French Mission and the other from the Portuguese Mission working together" on any kind of project (Robless and Sta. Maria n.d., 5).

14. The last two streets were named after Crighton, the British Resident Commissioner, and Kaartekoe, the Dutch commander who successfully laid siege to Malacca in 1641. The latter was quickly changed to Day Road, honoring another sympathetic British official. A village name, St. John's, was suggested by Fr. François at the same meeting. It never caught on. To this day the Settlement is known as the Portuguese Settlement in English,

Kampung Portugis or *Kampung Serani* ("Portuguese village" or "Christian village") in Malay, or *Padri să Chang* ("the Priests' Land") in Kristang.

15. The first *Regedor* (who served until 1938) was Felix Danker, father-in-law of future Settlement secretary George Bosco Lazaroo and grandfather of musician Joe Bosco Lazaroo. He built the first private house in the Settlement (No. 9 D'Albuquerque Road); with a raised porch and front portion, it was—until relatively recently—one of the grander houses in the Settlement.

16. The *branyo* is a flirtatious social dance in which couples advance and retreat but never touch. *Mata kantiga,* sung to the accompaniment of *branyo* music, is a duelling genre in which quatrains are exchanged between singers. Both will be discussed at length below. With the exception of language, *branyo* and *mata kantiga* are—today, at least—virtually interchangeable with the Malay genres *joget* and *dondang sayang,* respectively.

17. "compõe-se de 78 casas de madeira cobertas de folhas secas de palmeira—*attap*—para instalação de 557 descendentes de portugueses, na sua grande maioria pescadores ou pequenos funcionários" (Agência Geral do Ultramar 1954, 15).

By 1967, Chin Yik Poh counted 85 houses (64 government-built and 21 private). He observed a distinct division between the west and east halves of the Settlement (see map 2). The west half comprised 43 government and six private houses; the east half contained 21 government and 15 private houses (Chin 1967–68, 5). Of the houses built since 1967, only six were added to the west side, while 25 were built on the east side. Even today the difference remains apparent. Houses on the east side tend to be larger and more comfortable; residents are better off economically and have a larger proportion of white- than blue-collar jobs. The west side, in contrast, has a larger percentage of fishermen, manual laborers, and single breadwinners supporting larger families; lower educational achievements tend to perpetuate the status quo. Having often moved into the Settlement at a later date, some east-side residents do not count themselves (and are not counted by others) as real "Settlement people."

By June 1991, there were 117 houses in the Settlement, and, as there were only two more vacant lots, it is likely that this is close to the final count. At that time, the Settlement was home to 864 residents (450 male and 414 female). However, the total population is somewhat larger. In order to relieve severe overcrowding, a number of units were made available in government-built low-income apartment buildings just outside the Settlement boundary. By early 1991, 149 former Settlement residents (72 male and 77 female) had moved into 31 new apartments. In addition, 270 former residents (124 adults and 146 children) lived elsewhere in Malacca, and 122 single young people had moved away (primarily to Singapore or Kuala Lumpur) in order to find temporary work or to improve their job prospects (see Sarkissian 1993 for more detailed demographic analysis).

18. By 1967, only 12 out of 85 homes were without electricity because the householders could not afford the M$50.00 installation charge, even on a monthly payment scheme. The installation of water pipes was a more expensive proposition, costing up to M$300.00, depending on the distance of a residence from the main pipeline. Only 51 of the 85 houses had running water in 1967; the remainder relied on six public stand-pipes or on syphoning water from a neighbor's supply (Chin 1967–68, 38, 40).

19. Paul de Silva, the Settlement's fifth *Regedor,* served from 1953 until 1974. Michael Young served as *Regedor* from 1974 until he was succeeded by Peter Gomes in June 1998. By 1967 the Funeral Association boasted 65 members. Although the subscription rates were unchanged, the benefits had increased to M$75.00, or M$80.00 if the death occurred on a Sunday or public holiday (to cover overtime charges for the municipal hearse; Chin 1967–68, 42). There were 240 members by 1991. The entrance fee remains M$1.00 but the monthly subscription was increased to M$2.40; by 1991 funeral benefits stood at M$600 (Portuguese Settlement Funeral Association 1991).

20. The Zealanders were named in honor of a regiment from New Zealand stationed at Terendak Camp, a Commonwealth military base just outside town. The base was one of Malacca's major sources of employment during this period, and particularly close links developed between the Eurasians of the Settlement and the troops. In addition to several marriages, the link also resulted in books for schoolchildren, instruments for musicians, and visits from Santa Claus at Christmas. The closure of the base and departure of Commonwealth forces in 1969 led to a temporary economic depression in Malacca. Although the camp has since been reopened by the Malaysian army, it provides little in the way of employment for Settlement residents.

21. Other youth clubs have come and gone over the intervening years as different generations of socially active young people have formed their own clubs.

22. Inaugurated in February 1950, Sacred Heart Convent School was intended for children of the "poor fishermen" (Texeira 1961, 2:354). However, initial response from Settlement residents was so poor that the Sisters had "to visit homes in order to encourage parents to send their children to school" (B. Sta. Maria 1982, 134). In the end, Sacred Heart became a girls' school servicing the wider community; even today, there are few Settlement pupils.

23. Bernard Sta. Maria (1982, 133) adds that Lewis cited "Crown Land Rules as amended by Part XII of Scheduled [*sic*] of Transfer of Power Ordinance" as his legal precedent. The government memos are all reproduced in his younger brother's booklet on the development of the land title dilemma (J. Sta. Maria 1994, 24–27). I am not altogether convinced by Lewis's

memo of August 20, 1949 (ibid., 25); the typeface of the document looks more like an electric "golfball" type than anything that might have been found in 1949, and it omits the legal precedent quoted by Bernard.

24. State Grant 388, Lot 422, and Lot 549, respectively. The trade school was never built. As of August 1999, Lot 422 was still idle, although the government has allowed Settlement residents to use it as a sports field. In 1984, without formally repossessing the land, the government built a complex of restaurants called *Medan Portugis* (Malay: "Portuguese Square") and a car park on the site of their old playing field. Many residents still complain about this, describing the Square as a "white elephant" that has irreparably damaged community life. Now that the playing field is no longer in the center of the Settlement, residents say, spontaneous sports activities have ceased and parents can no longer keep watch on their children. Furthermore, they complain that the Square attracts undesirable locals who come to the Settlement to drink and often end up causing fights.

25. Bernard Sta. Maria, a Bandar Hilir resident and the only Portuguese Eurasian elected to the Malacca State Assembly, spent most of his political life campaigning on behalf of the Portuguese Settlement. In 1967, he founded the Portuguese Cultural Society (to be discussed below). After the 1969 general election, he turned his attention to politics, the land dispute, and improving the educational opportunities of Settlement children. Many of his projects, unfortunately, were hampered by lack of funding and opposition from the government. As a member of the opposition party, his political influence was not always of benefit to the Settlement. He died on July 30, 1987, at the height of the second lease controversy. His youngest brother, Joseph, has continued in his footsteps, both in the struggle for Settlement land rights and in the wider political forum. Joseph's 1994 booklet, *Undi Nos By Di Aki?* (Kristang: "Where Do We Go from Here?"), provides a detailed chronological account of the ongoing land dispute.

26. The conference was held in the Portuguese Settlement on February 19, 1995, and concluded with a press conference. Press coverage must have been excellent, for although my paper, "The Contribution of Portuguese Culture to Tourism in Malacca," was presented in absentia, it was soon quoted in a *Far Eastern Economic Review* feature (Hiebert 1995). The other papers were "The Linguistic Reflexes of the Historical Connections between the Malay and Portuguese Languages in the Malay World" (Alan Baxter, La Trobe University, Australia); "Kristang Family Heritage: Preliminary Remarks" (Brian O'Neill, Instituto Superior de Ciências do Trabalho e da Empresa, Lisbon); and "The Kristang G.I.S.: Community Planning and Empowerment using Geographical Information Systems" (Richard Dorall, Universiti Malaya). Two papers by local residents were also given: "Reclamation and the Settlement" (Michael Singho, Portuguese Settle-

ment) and "Leadership in the Portuguese Community" (Joseph St. Maria, Praya Lane). Of the three foreign-based scholars, only Alan Baxter was able to attend the conference in person. The collection of papers was published privately by Gerard Fernandis in 1998.

Chapter Two

1. Horace Sta. Maria (b. 1922) was one of the leading musical lights of the Malacca Eurasian community. With two other friends—Ernest Rodrigues (Ida's brother) and Camillo Gomes—he formed the Tres Amigos in 1947. The first, and perhaps most famous, Portuguese Eurasian singing group, the Tres Amigos started out singing "cowboy songs" but made a name for themselves with a few Portuguese songs and several Malay hits. Horace cites Jimmie Rodgers and Gene Autry among their musical influences. During the 1950s the group had regular live shows on Radio Malaya and a recording contract with HMV. Horace later taught high school in Malacca (at St. Francis Institute) before emigrating to Perth, Australia, in 1972. The Tres Amigos are still remembered with respect in Malaysian popular musical circles: in 1991 the "three men [who] won the hearts of the people and became the country's best known and most loved singing trio of the Fifties" were presented with an award by the Malaysian Country Music Association (*NST,* August 5, 1991).

2. Ida de Silva confirmed that the group was Fr. Pintado's idea, that the first dances were taught by a visiting friend of the priest, and that their initial repertoire was limited. Their costumes, sewn locally, were copied from book illustrations. Ida's husband, Clement, was the conductor-director, and she (by this time, one of the regular organists at St. Peter's) accompanied them on piano using staff notation from the same book (IRS, January 1, 1991). The visiting friend remained a mystery until Alan Baxter wrote the following: "I believe that the idea of teaching Portuguese regional dances was suggested to Padre Pintado by Ruy Cinatti, a Portuguese 'ethnologist' who lived in Timor and who visited Malacca" (pers. comm., July 12, 1999).

3. The *branyo,* the popular Settlement social dance, was performed by the "bride," the "bridegroom," and three pairs of dancers. The violinist on this occasion was Sylvester Nunis (Agência Geral do Ultramar 1954, 14–15).

4. Às 16.30, realizou-se no salão de dança do "Capitol" um chá oferecido pela Comunidade Portuguesa de Malaca, com exibição de danças e canções folclóricas. Assistiram cerca de 540 luso-descendentes, além de autoridades civis e militares, *leaders* das comunidades malaia, chinesa e indiana, bem como as personalidades de maior destaque de Malaca. Alguns dos luso-descendentes haviam percorrido mais de 70 milhas para assistir àquela reunião de homenagem a um Ministro da velha Pátria-Mãe (emphasis in original).

5. Complete program of the tea entertainment given in honor of Sarmento Rodrigues, May 19, 1952 (Agência Geral do Ultramar 1954, 22).

TEA ENTERTAINMENT: PROGRAMME

Portuguese National Hymn.

TEA

(A) Speech by Rev. Fr. M. J. Pintado.
  (a) Tiroliroliro—Dance.
(B) Speech by Mr. V. E. Dias J.P., C.H.
  (a) Amor mia Amor—Local Portuguese Song by Mr. Horace M. Sta. Maria.
  (b) Ala Banda Esti Banda by "Tres Amigos."
(C) Address by Mr. P. F. Pereira M.B.E.
  (a) Gingly Nona by "Tres Amigos."
  (b) Poesy "Qui Cause Bos Naqui Bem" by Mas. Emmanuel B. Lazaroo.
(D) Speech by the Honourable Resident Commissioner, Harold Georges [*sic*] Hammett.
  (a) "Until and Regresso ao Lar," by Mr. Clemente A. de Silva, accompanied by Mrs. C. A. de Silva.
(E) Reply by His Excellency the Commander Manuel Maria Sarmento Rodrigues, Minister for Portuguese Overseas Territories.
  (a) O Trevo (Trio) by Rodrigues Sisters
  (b) O Vira Vamos o Vira (Dance).
  (c) Saudade.

GOD SAVE THE QUEEN

6. Figure 5 (reproduced from Agência Geral do Ultramar 1954, facing p. 40) was taken at the May 19 performance. Clement de Silva is on the extreme left, wearing a suit and facing the group, Ida is standing in the back row on the left, and Ernest Rodrigues, Ivor Westerhout, and Jackie Lewis are the front three young men (left to right).

7. A dança portuguesa, "O tiroliroliro," executada por um grupo de rapazes e raparigas em trajes regionais portugueses. Este número despertou grande interesse e mereceu grandes aplausos pela elegância dos movimentos e pela graça dos trajes. . . . Continuou o programa com a dança popular "O Vira" aparecendo de novo o grupo dançante nos variegados e garriaos trajes regionais das províncias metropolitanas portuguesas.

8. Theodore Moissinac (b. 1912) was one of the few socially active Upper Tens not born and raised in Malacca. Born in Indonesia, he was educated in Penang and came to Malacca in 1936. He quickly became an active member of the local Eurasian musical scene, was elected Music Convenor of the Malacca Eurasian Volunteers, and held the post of choirmaster at St. Francis Xavier's church for over thirty years. He fought with the Volunteers

during World War II, was taken prisoner by the Japanese, and survived work on the death railway in Thailand (TM, July 31, 1991).

9. Christine Kanagarajah, née Rodrigues (b. 1936), was one of the younger members of the musically talented Rodrigues family. She left Malacca for Singapore after her marriage in 1958, but reactivated links with the dance groups after 1974 through her association with Fr. Sendim, a Portuguese priest posted to Singapore and later transferred to Malacca. For many years she visited Malacca periodically to teach Rancho Folclorico de San Pedro. Her regular visits became less frequent after her mother's death in 1982 and ceased after Fr. Sendim's death in a 1989 road accident. At the time of our conversation she taught music at St. Anthony's Convent School, Singapore. Since she is still known around the Settlement as Christie Rodrigues (rather than Kanagarajah), I will henceforth use her maiden name.

10. Christie Rodrigues remembered the dances being "Fara Pera," "Ti' Anika," "Vira Atra Pasados," and "Baté Peo" (CRK, March 19, 1991). Ida Rodrigues remembered "Verde Gaio" being one of the first taught dances with "Anda Roda" and "Kamasha" coming from the book (IRS, January 1, 1991). Neither sister could remember the author or title of the book. Christie described it as a small booklet containing the music and steps of four dances. Ida said it contained descriptions and illustrations of typical costumes, including footwear and the hanging pocket commonly worn by girls from the Minho region. Lucile Armstrong's 1948 booklet, *Dances of Portugal,* comes closest to their combined description: it contains a section on costumes (with an illustration of the hanging pocket) and includes the music and steps for four dances, "A Rosa," "Paderinha," "Vira Extrapassado," and "Vira." Two of these pieces, "Paderinha" (or "Baté Peu," as it has become known in Malacca) and "Vira Extrapassado" (or "Vira Atra Passados") were on Christie's list. The other two "Vira" ("O Vira Vamos") and "A Rosa" were both known and danced by the group at that time according to Ida. If this is indeed the book in question, Christie may simply have misremembered which pieces she learned from it almost forty years ago. Since Armstrong (1948, 40) mentions "an extreme scarcity of notated Portuguese dances in published form," it is unlikely that there were many other such books available at the time. That it was found in a small bookstore in Malacca is not surprising. Still in the same location (on Riverside Street, a stone's throw from Christ Church, the Clock Tower, and St. Paul's Hill) and run by the now ancient Mr. Lim, Lim's Bookstore remains the best place in Malacca to find unusual books connected with local history and culture.

11. Arthur Sta. Maria had a similar opportunity to visit Portugal in 1968. Although Arthur had already decided to emigrate to Australia by that point, Fr. Pintado felt he had earned the trip (sponsored by the Portuguese government) for all the work he had done with the dance group in Malacca. He

attended a folk festival in the city of Viseu in central Portugal. According to Arthur, the folk festival "was held every August in connection with a festival of the stripping of the corn. . . . There were lots of songs and dances. I saw all the dances—all the ones we did in Malacca were quite authentic [he is referring here to the music]. The way we do the dances in Malacca, however, was more 'gentle.' " Arthur emigrated to Perth, Australia, in 1972 (pers. comm., June 21, 1999).

12. Figure 7, courtesy of Patrick de Silva, shows the first all-Settlement group. Back row (left to right): William Tan, Domingos de Costa, John de Costa, George de Costa (Dom's brother), Norman de Mello, Aloysius de Mello, Patrick de Silva. Front: Theresa and Elizabeth Sequerah (twins), George Bosco Lazaroo, Arthur Sta. Maria, Paul de Silva (*Regedor* and Patrick's father), Flora de Costa, and Magdeline Sta. Maria.

Figure 8, courtesy of Aloysius Sta. Maria, shows the same group performing at the *padang* (Malay: "field") opposite St. Francis Institute. The only dancers who can be identified clearly are Domingos de Costa and Magdeline Sta. Maria (Aloy's sister) on the left side and Norman de Mello in the center (ASM, June 24, 1991).

13. Complete program of the Christmas concert performed in the Sacred Heart Convent school hall, Portuguese Settlement, circa 1953 (Lazaroo ca. 1953).

1. Overture (Tai pun, O Tiroliroliro, and Seti Semanas)
2. Merry Christmas, Silent Night, Ala Marinheiros, Vira (Dance)
3. O Amor Eu Nunca mandar com vos vai (solo by Norman de Mello)
4. Won't you buy my pretty flowers (girls)
5. O Malao (quartet)
6. Gingle Bells—Selections by Mr. Dennis Pestana
7. Os Marinheiros—O Vira (Dance)
8. Union is strength (Boys)
9. Doggie in the Window (Trio)
10. My Pretty Maid
11. Bom Bom Filha (solo by Noel Felix)
12. Rhythm of the Islands (solo by Roosevelt de Costa—Jula Jula [*sic*] dance)
13. The Prodigal (boys)
14. A Portuguese song (solo)
15. Ti-a-nica (choir), O verde gaio (Dance)
16. The Clown (selections by Mr. Dennis Pestana)
17. The Unusual Star (girls)
18. 25 years R. I.
19. O-Limao—O Malao (Dance)
20. Branho (Local folk dance) (N. de Mello and N. Felix sing)
21. Review of Portuguese songs followed by Adeste Fideles

GOD SAVE THE QUEEN

14. Complete program of the concert performed in the Sacred Heart Convent school hall, Portuguese Settlement, on June 29, 1956, for the Festa di San Pedro (Lazaroo 1956).

    1. Os Marinheiros and Ala Marinheiros (Portuguese Settlement Youths)
    2. Selection of Portuguese Songs (Portuguese Settlement Catholic Youths Harmonica Band)
    3. Balarico, Ti Anica de Lowlay, and O Trevo (Tres Cavalieros)
    4. The Vira (Dance)
    5. Denny Pestana, the Clown
    6. Allegria and another Portuguese song (Horace Sta. Maria)
    7. Sete Semanas (Youths)
    8. O Limao (Dance)
    9. Denny Pestana, clown
   10. O Malao and Tiro-Liro-Liro (Dances)
   11. Branyo (Denny Pestana & the boys will invite the guests to dance)
   12. Saudade

GOD SAVE THE QUEEN

15. Freddie James Scully (1933–94) was the son of Frederick John Scully, the performer of Hawaiian songs and "Pack Up Your Troubles" at the 1933 Malacca Volunteers' variety concert. Walter Sequerah, brother of Cyril (the first PSYC President) and of Elizabeth and Theresa (twins who had been among the earliest Settlement dancers), later married Marianne Lazaroo and became Joe's brother-in-law.

16. This move from a literate to an oral tradition is not as singular as it might at first appear. In fact, similar processes have occurred in other "folk revival" traditions. For example, as Alyn Shipton observed, "I think there's a parallel here with the English folksong and dance tradition. When I interviewed Martin Carthy, he said he learned his songs from sheet music by Vaughan Williams and Grainger and now people learn from him" (pers. comm., March 2, 1996; see also Feintuch 1993).

17. Since census statistics include Portuguese Eurasians in the undifferentiated category of "Others" (i.e., not Malay, Chinese, or Indian), accurate population statistics are hard to ascertain. In the 1980 census the population of the entire state of Malacca was 464,754 (87,494 of whom lived within the limits of Malacca Town) of which only 0.7 percent or 3,247 persons were classified as "Others." Although the population of the entire state had increased by 1990 to 504,502 persons, it is unlikely that the percentage of "Others" had changed much.

18. Noel Felix (b. 1932) already had a reputation as a good singer when he left the Settlement to join the army in 1951. After being discharged in 1958 he returned to Malacca and joined the water department, where he remained until he retired. Although away from the Settlement during the

crucial early period, Felix learned the songs and dances from Arthur Sta. Maria. As Arthur reminisced, "since he couldn't read very well at that time, he learned everything by heart" (pers. comm., June 21, 1999). Noel also began to compose songs himself. He led Bernard Sta. Maria's Portuguese Cultural Society dance group, and continues to lead the group, now re-named Tropa de Malaca (NF, July 17, 1990). Today Noel not only reads well, but reads fast. In the space of about three days, he read this entire manuscript and provided several useful clarifications.

19. In fact, both *joget* and *branyo* share the same underlying three-against-two rhythm, and melodies may be interchanged at will. *Mata kantiga* and *dondang sayang* both share the same poetic structure (four-line *pantun* verses), though not the same accompanying rhythm. By switching from Kristang to Malay and from a *branyo* tune and beat to the *dondang sayang* melody and distinctive rhythm, the best *mata kantiga* singers could easily adapt to the Malay duelling form. See chapter 4 for further discussion of these genres.

Chapter Three

1. In this chapter the ethnographic present refers to the situation as it existed between 1990 and 1992, at the height of the tourist boom.

2. While Christmas and Easter remain important religious occasions for the general Catholic community, more "folkloric" celebrations (such as feast days of locally important saints) have proved more acceptable subjects for incorporation into the government-approved national calendar. This tour-ism-driven calendar attempts to celebrate national diversity while down-playing sensitive non-Malay (i.e., non-Islamic) religious holy days (see Sarkissian 1999). Since the feast of St. Peter, patron saint of fishermen, quickly became associated with the Portuguese Settlement, the Praya Lane community adopted the feast of St. John (San Juang, in Kristang), and the Penang Eurasian community adopted the feast of St. Anne. Although all communities observe each feast day privately, they tend to "specialize" in one to maximize the profit that can be made from drawing a large number of tourists and from government sponsorship.

3. When Freddie Scully started his new group, some members of other groups accused him of stealing their music and choreography, of being in essence, a copycat. *Tiru* in Malay, literally means "to copy"; *tukang tiru-tiru* means "one who copies" (i.e., a "copycat"). But since *tiru* was also a Kristang word (a noun meaning "a shot"), Scully decided to use the intended slur as the name for his group. The initial "D'," though ungrammatical, makes the name sound "more Portuguese." The name Strela di Melaka, in con-trast, makes an explicit political statement. By using the Malay spelling "Melaka" instead of the Portuguese "Malaca" (as in Tropa de Malaca) or the English "Malacca," the organizer (George Alcantra) emphasized his

alliance with the ruling government party and with the local state assembly-man, Datuk Gan Boon Leong.

4. Choreography became a particularly sensitive issue for Tropa de Malaca dancers after the formation of Strela di Melaka. Since the latter (led by ex-Tropa de Malaca dancers) adopted their choreography wholesale, Tropa de Malaca dancers have created new variations to make their dances more complex. The significance of this new choreography cannot be underestimated: it is the first example of an organic creative process in operation (rather than the rote reproduction of fixed combinations).

5. Unlike the situation in any of the other groups, the leader (Scully) and his two chief musicians (Georgie de Costa and Andrew Carvalho) are all roughly the same age. The most talented musician in the group, Andrew Carvalho is competent on guitar and keyboards when necessary but usually plays violin or ukulele. Although the violin was a common Portuguese Eurasian instrument in the past, Carvalho is the only violinist in any of the dance groups today. Significantly, however, his mastery of the violin comes not from playing the traditional Portuguese-Eurasian *branyo* but from his background as a country-western musician. Now in his sixties, Andrew came from an Upper Tens family and grew up in the Bandar Hilir area with the Sta. Maria and Rodrigues boys. Andrew was one of the original Tres Amigos (with Horace Sta. Maria and Ernest Rodrigues) but left the group before it became famous. Forsaking his growing reputation as a musician and song writer, Andrew left Malacca for Singapore in 1951 to train as a teacher. Even so, he is still remembered in the music business and was honored with a Country Western Association Hall of Fame Award for pioneering country music in Malaysia (*NST,* December 19, 1990).

6. This privilege was extended to me as a temporary, but equal, member of the group. Unlike my experience as a (relatively) obedient, silent member of Rancho Folclorico San Pedro, I was expected to voice an opinion and contribute to communal decision making at Tropa de Malaca group meetings.

7. In September 1990, an international group of photographers visited Malaysia to shoot pictures for a book, *A Day in the Life of Malaysia.* Dominic Sansoni, a Eurasian photojournalist from Columbo, Sri Lanka, arranged a photo shoot with Joe and Rancho Folclorico San Pedro in the ruined Dutch fort on St. John's Hill. Performing elsewhere with Tropa de Malaca, I was unable to attend the shoot but gave my camera to M. Veera Pandiyan, a local journalist, and asked him to take as many pictures as he could. The poses Sansoni arranged clearly illustrate his romanticized vision of the "lost Portuguese." In figure 10, dancers (left to right) are Edmund Lazaroo, James Sebastian, Elaine Lazaroo, and Juana Lai; musicians (left to right) are Gerry Fernandis (accordion), Joe Lazaroo (guitar), Francis "Sub" de Costa (guitar), and (almost obscured) Basil Bournaparte (tambor).

8. By July 1996, Joe said his regular price for a single show in Kuala Lumpur was M$2,800. He charges less for shows closer to home: after a recent single performance in Port Dickson (a coastal town on the Malacca side of Kuala Lumpur), for example, he was able to give each musician and dancer M$80. As he said, with a big smile on his face and a shrug of his shoulders, "if they pay, we give them a good show; if no money, we don't go" (JBL, July 14, 1996).

9. Noel's son, Nolan, was the first student from the less affluent west side of the Settlement to attend university. He studied accounting at Universiti Malaya and graduated in spring 1990. His expenses were partially defrayed by a scholarship from the Portuguese Settlement Development Board (a fund set up by a wealthy Eurasian property developer, Datuk Eugene Campos), and partially by sponsorship from a Kuala Lumpur bank. Unable to find a suitable position within the bank when he graduated, Nolan returned to Malacca and got a job locally as an auditor. Now married, he lives with his parents, is busy raising a family, and supplements his income by tutoring Settlement youngsters. Noel's youngest daughter, Sally, married a visiting tourist and now lives in Germany.

10. As is the case with many company bands in Malacca, a large number of the musicians are Portuguese Eurasians, mostly from the Settlement. In 1991, for example, the Tenaga Nasional band comprised Gerard de Costa (guitar), Charlie Sta. Maria (guitar), Bob Moissinac (vocals/guitar/keyboards), Francis Theseira (saxophone), Laura de Mello (vocals), Hock (a Chinese married to a Praya Lane Portuguese woman; drums), and two Malays. Gerard's sister-in-law, Laura, was the only member of the band not employed by Tenaga Nasional. Charlie Sta. Maria, a former Rancho Folclorico San Pedro musician, also played occasionally for his father-in-law, Stephen Theseira. Bob Moissinac is a son of Theodore, St. Francis Xavier in the 1953 pageant.

11. To add a further strand of complexity to the web, I am Jeremy's godmother.

Chapter Four

1. Residents are using the word "music" very broadly here to encompass the melodies, associated texts, and choreography of dances as well as the melodies and associated texts of songs. The waters are further muddied when a dance tune and text performed without choreography is reclassified as a song (e.g., "Vira di Bairu Português," normally a choreographed dance, is sometimes performed as a song by Joe Lazaroo). The opposite, adding choreography to what is usually a song, rarely happens.

2. These tables, which focus on the relatively stable dance repertoire, include all the dances performed between 1990 and 1992 by Tropa de Malaca, Rancho Folclorico San Pedro, Tropa de Assunta (Praya Lane), and D'Tiru-Tiru; I have omitted the shortest-lived of the groups, Strela di Melaka, on

the grounds that it did not exist long enough to develop a distinctive repertoire. Songs, interspersed for the sake of variety or to give the dancers a
rest, are drawn from a much larger floating corpus that will be discussed
separately below.

3. Thus, for example, Freddie Scully could argue that D'Tiru-Tiru's core
   dances were "more authentic" than those of Tropa de Malaca because
   Georgie de Costa (a member of the first Settlement group) was the lead
   musician and dance instructor of D'Tiru-Tiru. It did not seem to matter
   that Georgie had formerly been a member of Tropa de Malaca and, according to Noel Felix, had copied Tropa de Malaca's choreography.

4. Two dances—"The Portuguese Washerwoman" and "Korradinyo"—stand
   out as exceptions to this general statement. The former has always been
   something of an oddity in the repertoire (see table 1, note a). The latter,
   originally one of the four melodies learned from Armstrong's book (where
   it is identified as "A Rosa," a *corridinho* from Oliveira do Hospital in the
   Beira region), was rechoreographed by Christie Rodrigues after 1974 and
   is now performed only by Rancho Folclorico San Pedro. For this reason,
   it should more properly be grouped with the post-1974 repertoire.

5. Copied from videotapes and cassettes sent as gifts by Portuguese tourists,
   these dances are the only examples of a Settlement resident taking the initia-
   tive in acquiring new material; they have not been performed since D'Tiru-
   Tiru was disbanded in 1994.

6. Songs from this period include "Ala Marinheiros," "Alecrim," "Indu Eu,"
   "Os Marinheiros," "Pico Pico Serenico," "Ravela Nos Namoricas" (or "Na
   roda duma fugeira"), "Romaria" (or "Tangem os Sinos"), "Saudade," "Sete
   Semanas," "O Trevo," and "Verdi Gaio."

7. Noel Felix's compositions include "O Bela" (Old woman), "Floris yo kubisá" (Flower that I admire), and "Kantu sen fazé fabor" (A few cents to
   please you). In addition to newly composed songs, Noel also sings popular
   songs with Kristang lyrics: for example, "O Maria" is a cover version of
   "Isle of Capri"; "El Bayo," which uses the same melody as Tropa de Assunta's dance, "Alegrá," and "Suku suku" are thought to be set "Spanish"
   tunes, but their original models have been long forgotten. Joe Lazaroo's
   compositions include "Dia di San Pedro" (Saint Peter's day), "Kristang di
   Padri să Chang" (People of the Portuguese Settlement), "Cantar" (Sing),
   and "Malacca."

8. Theseira has set Kristang lyrics to a wide range of melodies, both Western
   and Malay. Those regularly performed by Tropa de Assunta include "Floris
   bramilu" (Red flower), "Marinyeros feradu" (Drunken sailors), and "Prispi
   di ela" (The prince over there). Like the texts of his dances, many of his
   lyrics draw upon the imagery and language found in *mata kantiga* verses.

9. The six songs are "Asi-să Macau" (That's Macau!), "Mama-să filu" (Mama's
   boy), "Macau, terra minha" (Macau, my country), "Nhum Careca" (The

bald man), "Longi di terra amado" (Far from my beloved country), which Noel renders as "Lonzi di tera matu" (Far from the jungle), and "Aqui Bobo" (Here's the clown). All appear on the Tuna Macaense CD *Macau Să Assi* (Tuna Macaense 1994).

10. Joe's favorites include "O Cochicho" (The whistle), "Coimbra" (also called "April in Portugal"), "Fado de Coimbra" (also called "Coimbra Rio Mundego"), "Vinyo verde" (Green wine), and, less commonly, "A fonte de minha aldeia" (At my village fountain), "Chapeu preto" (Black hat), "Lisboa antiga" (Old Lisbon), "Uma Casa Portuguesa" (A Portuguese House), and "Minha mae" (My mother). Noel's standard songs include "Asi-să Macau" (That's Macau!), "Mama-să filu" (Mama's boy), and "Vinyo verde." Many of these "evergreens" have been popular in Portugal since the early 1950s. Several of these songs (e.g., "Coimbra," "Uma Casa Portuguesa," and "Lisboa Antiga") were recorded by the famous Portuguese singer Amália Rodrigues in 1952.

11. The cassette contained six songs and five instrumental numbers (see note 9). The liner insert included the song lyrics and instrumental titles but nothing else: no information about performers or date of publication. The cover picture juxtaposed images that would not have looked out of place on a cassette entitled "Malacca": a Portuguese tombstone, a cannon in the foreground with a red headscarf draped over it, and a *fado* guitar leaning against the cannon. The music was performed by an unidentified local *tuna* band. Traditionally, *tunas* were amateur string bands formed by Macanese students to play at Carnival and other street processions. The mostly portable instruments include mandolins, guitars, ukulele, and sometimes violin; for indoor performances, however, a large drum and string bass are often added. Today, *tuna* ensembles in Macau are generally semiprofessional (dos Santos Ferreira 1994).

12. I discovered this tidbit soon after returning from Malacca in 1991 thanks to the Brazilian ethnomusicologist Samuel Araujo (then a fellow graduate student at the University of Illinois), who recognized it while we were playing music together one Saturday night. The Macanese text is similar to that of the Brazilian original, the only significant difference being the change of title from "Mama Eu Quero" (I want my Mama) to "Mama-să Filu" (Mama's boy). The original song, "Mama Eu Quero" was published by Robbins Music Corp. in 1939. Words and music were by Jararaca Paiva and Vincente Paiva.

13. I am grateful to Marlene Wong for the discographical information.

14. I am grateful to William Seigh, who remembered this scene, and to *I Love Lucy* fan Jonathan Angus of West Virginia, who identified the episode and provided a videotape.

15. The final vowel of "Tia," "Aunty," is usually lost in the elision with "Anika," "Annie."

16. Alportel, another place mentioned in João do Rio's 1909 version of the text, is also located in the same region.

17. "Ti' Anika" is still well known in Brazil, according to Samuel Araujo. It also appears on a cassette of Portuguese string band music from Hawai'i sent to me by another colleague, Andrew Weintraub. Finally, according to Ida de Silva, it is one of the dances performed by a dance group established by the Malacca-Portuguese community of Perth, Australia.

18. There is one context in which "Ti' Anika" is performed off-stage in the Settlement: small children imitating their older siblings sometimes dance in circles, singing its melody. While I was learning the dance repertoire, I spent many hours each day practicing accordion in a shady spot under the mango tree in my front yard. One of my neighbors, Flora Felix (Noel Felix's sister-in-law), told me that her three-year-old granddaughter waited expectantly each morning until I got to "Ti' Anika." As soon as I struck up the tune, Christina began to "practice" the dance in her front yard several houses down the road. Once she mastered her own version of the dance, Christina formed a mini dance group and began to direct other small cousins.

19. Briged Seni Negeri Melaka is translated by local residents as "Malacca State Cultural Brigade." Strictly speaking, however, the Malay word "*seni*" refers to "arts" in general rather than to "culture" (Malay: "*kebudayaan*"). For a lengthier discussion of this particular cultural troupe, see Sarkissian 1998a.

20. I would like to thank my friend, Puan Ramah Arshad of Ampang Jaya, Kuala Lumpur, for sharing the videotape of the Sri Inai Junior School concert.

21. Alan Baxter has suggested that *minya* might date from the nineteenth century, when Portuguese and colloquial Portuguese were taught by the Catholic Mission and by the London Missionary Society (pers. comm. July 12, 1999).

22. Philip Thomas (1986, 15) has shown that *dondang sayang* is a complex poetical genre in which several different layers of meaning coexist: a good quatrain has a surface-level direct meaning, a middle-level metaphorical meaning, and a deep-level abstract meaning. Although there is little recognition of deeper meaning in *mata kantiga* quatrains today, it is not clear whether the genre was poetically more sophisticated in the past. I have noted only one instance in which a Settlement resident attributed deeper meaning to two particular quatrains, suggesting that they referred to the time of Dutch persecution (refugees spreading information in the first verse, trying to escape in the second):

Putu mayang kenti kenti	The rice-flour cake is very hot
Suá koku ja laras	The coconut has been ground fine
Ubi nobǎs di Malacca	I heard news from Malacca
Albi koku ja rakuá	The coconut palm has been uprooted

Barku San José	The ship "San José"
Lantá bela botá kuré	Raises sail, ready to run
Fila mina nă rentu kama	The virgin girl in her bed
Baté korpu keré muré	Beats her body, wants to die

The opinion of the resident in question, Gerard Fernandis, may, however, be anomalous. The son of an upper-class Eurasian who moved into the Settlement and owns one of the large houses on its periphery, Jerry is one of the few Settlement residents to have gone on to higher education (including a Gulbenkian Foundation scholarship to study in Portugal).

23. In fact, Fernando makes a far better job of transcribing the melodic rhythm than did Silva Rêgo (1941, 225), when he transcribed the Malaccan version. By notating the melody in compound duple time with a ♩ ♪ ♪ ♩ rhythmic pattern, Fernando almost captures the characteristic, unruly triplet-duplet rhythmic underpinning. Silva Rêgo, in contrast, manages to put a lively tune into a straightjacket by notating it in a regular simple duple time (♩. ♪ ♩ ♩). In addition, he made the mistake of using a G major key signature even though his melody was clearly transcribed in C major.

24. For a discussion of other types of cultural show in Malaysia, see Sarkissian 1998a.

25. In fact, producing the compact disc *Kantiga di Padri să Chang* proved to be a challenging experience. In the end, the Portuguese ethnomusicologist Susana Sardo managed to work backwards from my Settlement versions of Portuguese songs to piece together Portuguese versions which we then translated into English. When I gave Noel Felix a copy of the disc, he read the English translation of the first track (his version of the song "Sekush marinyeros"), looked at me with a big grin on his face, and said "so that's what the song's about!"

26. Both versions differ substantially from the earliest published text I have found, which appears in a 1909 collection compiled by João do Rio and published in Brazil. In this version, each verse gives Auntie Annie a different home town (Loulé, Fuseta, Aljezur, and Alportel) and refers to a different item of clothing (a muffler, a black skirt, a blue skirt, and a cloak).

27. In translating *bara preta* as "east side," it is possible that Noel is thinking of the Malay words, *barat* ("west") and *praia* ("coast").

28. There are only two changes: one approximation (*perapus* for *ferrapos)* and one substitution (*saia* for *camisa*). *Saia* and *camisa* are both Portuguese words for items of clothing, but the former is used in the Settlement and the latter is not. Even the title has been subject to domestication: since *fara* has no meaning in Kristang but *perá* (or *sperá*) means "to wait," the title is often rendered as "Fala Pera" or "Fala Spera" (Kristang: "[he/she] says [to] wait").

29. I suspect that this smoothing-out of movements has been happening for a while. In describing his visit to a folk festival in Portugal in 1968, Arthur Sta. Maria commented that although the dances were "authentic" (and here he is referring to the musical accompaniment), the way they performed the dances in Malacca was more "gentle" (pers. comm., June 21, 1999). It was only when Christie Rodrigues decided to choreograph dances based on what she had seen in Portugal that the sharper, tighter style was introduced.

30. The Malay word *pantun* refers to a complex four-line poetic genre, which among other things forms the basis of the *dondang sayang* (see Philip Thomas 1986). In this conversation, Noel uses *pantun* as a verb, meaning "to make up verses." That he uses a Malay word to describe this process reinforces the hybridity of the tradition.

31. *Potra* is the common Kristang pronunciation of the Portuguese *porta,* "door."

32. *Menggaring* is a Malay verb from the stem *garing,* "crisp." *Rosa menggaring* (lit., "crisped rose") is the Malay term for jasmine flower.

33. Silva Rêgo (1941, 53) interprets this quatrain differently: "A afeição tem tal poder sôbre o homem que, por amor da mulher, é capaz de se matar" (Love has such power over man that, for the love of a woman, he is capable of suicide; my translation).

34. Alor Gajah is one of the three major towns in the state of Malacca. The other two are Malacca Town and Jasin.

35. Silva Rêgo gives the following variant (1941, 29):

Passá nona sa porta	As I was passing your door
Sepatu gritá gritá	Wearing tap-dancing shoes
Salada botá na mesa	Put a salad on the table
Tudo gente cobiçá	Everyone admired it

36. To give an example (romanized words are Malay, not Kristang):

O Nona, minya Nona	O Nona, my Nona
Yo tã bendé kacang putih	I'm selling white peanuts
Agora sã fila fila	Girls nowadays
Tã kuré kú orang putih	Are running after white men's asses

37. One other tune, simply called *branyo,* is occasionally used in conjunction with scolding verses that begin with the formula "Ala banda ku isti banda." Settlement musicians are not sure whether this melody is an example of one of the *branyo* subtypes or not.

38. Baxter's field tapes are probably the only recorded examples of the old-style *branyo.* According to Noel Felix, this particular tune (which he calls

a fast *bintana*) should be accompanied not by the characteristic triplet-duplet *branyo* rhythm, but by a running sixteenth-note pattern played on *tambor*, which he described as a small, shallow double-headed cylindrical drum played with two sticks. Although Noel's drummer, Benjamin de Costa described the *tambor* as "Malay," no indigenous drum fits his description. It is likely, then, that Noel and 'Amin are both referring to a European-style military side drum, an assumption supported by the sound of the drum on Baxter's recording. The use of side-drum coupled with the military-style rhythm, both unique to this single item of repertoire, might suggest a last vestige of Portuguese (or at least, European) influence. 'Amin's assumption that the *tambor* is Malay further suggests a long-standing absorption into the local music scene.

Chapter Five

1. Festivals of this sort are, as Kirshenblatt-Gimblett (1998, 59) has observed, the perfect entrée for tourists "who have difficulty deciphering and penetrating the quotidian of their destination. . . . Public and spectacular, [they] have the practical advantage of offering in a concentrated form, at a designated time and place, what the tourist would otherwise search out in the diffuseness of everyday life, with no guarantee of ever finding it."

2. One other wedding scene was performed during Malacca Tourism Week 1991. Although it demonstrated ethnically Malay traditions, the Malacca Malay Wedding received much less publicity, was held at Taman Mini Malaysia in the suburb of Ayer Keroh, and only merited a midweek afternoon time slot.

3. It is worth remembering that Sarmento Rodrigues's visit to the Portuguese Settlement on May 19, 1952 was celebrated with a "traditional wedding scene." Significantly, although the two performances were given almost exactly forty years apart, George Bosco Lazaroo was the narrator on both occasions.

4. The procession, the seating of bride and groom at a dais, and the receiving of guests are features common to traditional Malay, Chitty Melaka (Straits-born Indian), and Portuguese-Eurasian wedding celebrations despite their respectively Muslim, Hindu, and Christian religious underpinnings. Although there are marked similarities between the wedding processions of all three groups, each retains its own distinctive musical accompaniment: Malay processions are heralded by an ensemble of *kompang* (frame drums of Middle Eastern origin) of different sizes that play rhythmically interlocking patterns; Chitty Melaka processions are led by one or more South Indian *nagaswaram* (large oboe-type instrument) and *tavil* (double-headed barrel-shaped drum); and in former times, according to old photographs, Portuguese Eurasian processions were accompanied by a hybrid ensemble comprising violins, small hand-held gong, and *rebana* (another type of Malay-style frame drum).

5. Breaks of this sort are a practical necessity, especially when performing outdoors during the daytime. Even when the sun has gone down and the evening temperature is somewhat cooler, the tropical humidity still makes physical exertion in full costume uncomfortable and tiring. In addition to these general moments of rest, the practice of alternating personnel between one dance and the next insures that individual dancers are rested and everyone gets a turn to perform.

6. He does not quite succeed. He interrupts his father's narration at one point to announce the title of a song (his own composition), "Vira di Bairu Português."

7. Bosco prepares and types out all his speeches in advance, hence the unusually florid language. Since he saves his typescripts and reuses the same material repeatedly, it is not inconceivable that parts of this text were used in 1952 when he narrated a similar wedding scene for Sarmento Rodrigues's visit.

8. Western-style suits are not the only markers of non-Portuguese European identity. The *kronchi,* the mitre-shaped decoration hung over the front door and the door to the bridal room, is a vestige of Dutch wedding "coronets" or *kroontje* (see time index 32.43 in the table). According to McGilvray (1982, 250), this was the only identifiable Dutch custom maintained by upper-class Burghers of Sri Lanka.

9. "Vira di Sta. Marta" is the Settlement version of the famous *vira* from the town of Santa Marta do Portuzelo. A large village close to the city of Viana do Castelo on the northwestern coast (in the Minho region), Santa Marta do Portuzelo has one of the oldest and best-known folkloric groups in the country (Salwa El-Shawan, pers. comm., September 5, 1997).

10. This is one of only two dance pieces in the Settlement repertoire that includes a modulation. The other piece, "Asas Brancas," another Sendim-Rodrigues dance performed only by Rancho Folclorico San Pedro, is the most technically difficult piece in the musical repertoire and is rarely performed.

11. "Tiru Liru Liru" was a favorite of Freddie Scully's group, D'Tiru-Tiru—one of Scully's most enduring catch phrases being, "here's 'Tiru Liru Liru' D'Tiru-Tiru for you!" Strangely, it is one of the few examples of "our music" not performed by Noel Felix's group, Tropa de Malaca. As an item in Rancho Folclorico San Pedro's repertoire, however, it is uncharacteristic: the simplicity of the choreography (comprising hand motions and turning on the spot) is at odds with their energetic and virtuosic style. Of course, this simplicity makes it the ideal audience-participation dance.

12. This is not always the case, however. When performing a longer show, Joe Lazaroo uses a combination of older dances (e.g., "Ti' Anika," "Anda Roda,' etc.), Fr. Sendim-era Portuguese songs, and his own songs to fill out the middle order of the program.

13. "Lisboa antiga," by José Galhardo, Amadeu do Vale, and Raul Portela, was recorded by Rodrigues in 1952. Tropa de Malaca wedding scenes diverge from the Rancho Folclorico San Pedro model at this point. Instead of playing soft background music to accompany the distribution of cake and wine, Noel Felix complicates the synthesis still further by staging a short entertainment—a cultural dance show—for the wedding party and their onstage tourist guests. Temporal and spatial distances collapse as dancers in Portuguese costume, representing the imagined, mythical world of D'Albuquerque, perform simultaneously for the wedding party in *kebaya kompridu* and suits, representing the hybridized, old-time world of the Settlement, the transformed tourist guests in their privileged position on stage, and the real audience watching in the Square.

14. Joe "Bomba" Lazaroo passed away in October 1999.

15. Theresa de Costa passed away on January 13, 1998.

Chapter Six

1. See www.geocities.com/TheTropics/Paradise/9221 for the web site of the Malacca Portuguese Eurasian Association.

2. This phase of the dispute follows two earlier reclamation projects in the area. The first, now the site of a huge new commercial subdivision called Malacca Raya, was completed in the mid-1980s; the second, completed in the mid-1990s, is the site of a new shopping mall (Mahkota Parade), a large private hospital, and several blocks of condominiums. In addition to landlocking the old Praya Lane community, the reclamation seriously affected prawn fishing from the Portuguese Settlement. In addition to destroying plankton and thus prawn breeding and spawning grounds, it also led to a build-up of silt that made wading for prawns using butterfly-shaped nets (called *langgiang*) extremely difficult.

3. Pulau Melaka, a ten-year, RM$2 billion project contracted by Inno-Enhance Sdn. Bhd., is already under construction. An estimated 90 hectares (225 acres) will be reclaimed for bungalow lots, condominiums, shop lots, a marina, a water theme park, and recreational picnic areas; one-sixth of this prime real estate will be given to the state government. The artificially created islands will be connected to the mainland by two 350 meter bridges (*The Sun,* July 5, 1996 and July 7, 1996). The second project, undertaken by Olympia Land Bhd., will reclaim 140 hectares (350 acres) along two miles of the Portuguese Settlement and Ujong Pasir coastline on which a self-contained township comprising offices, condominiums, a hotel, private colleges, and a theme park will be built (*Sunday Star,* August 7, 1994).

4. The Fishermen's Action Committee gained a good deal of press coverage, forcibly bringing their plight to the attention of the public. For example, with national attention focused on Malacca during the annual Festa di San Pedro, Danker and about fifty fishermen staged a peaceful demonstration

outside the offices of Inno-Enhance Sdn. Bhd. Carrying a coffin to symbol-ize the death of their livelihood, Danker and his cohorts accused the devel-opers of reneging on their promise to compensate six fishermen whose nets had been damaged and to provide initial compensation to the fishermen for loss of livelihood (*The Star,* June 26, 1996).

5. As was mentioned in the technical notes, Kristang is an oral language. It is rarely used as a written medium of communication within the Settle-ment. Most public announcements are thus written in English, the pre-ferred lingua franca of the Settlement. Occasional announcements written in Malay are rarely read by older members of the community.

6. See Sarkissian 1999 for a more detailed comparison of religious and secular festivals in the Settlement.

7. The *Irmang di Greza* is an all-male para-religious confraternity founded in 1553 by the Dominican Fr. Gaspar de Cruz. The *Irmang di Greza* still play a role (particularly at Eastertide) in the two Portuguese Mission estab-lishments, St. Peter's Church and Assumption Chapel (Baxter 1987, 21).

8. The fishermen's refusal to participate in the folkloric aspect of the festival (the boat-decorating contest) but their desire, nevertheless, to have their boats blessed suggests that although the Festa di San Pedro has acquired new meaning for its producers through commoditization to the extent that "what used to be a religiously meaningful ritual for an internal public, [has] become a culturally significant self-representation before an external public" (Cohen 1988, 382), this is not the whole story. Under the veneer of commercialism, the religious meaning still remains. Although many of the decorated boats no longer sail, for those that do, the priest's blessing is real.

9. Amanah Saham Nasional is a government savings bond scheme open to *bumiputras,* or ethnic Malays, but not to Malaysians of other ethnic back-grounds (Chinese, Indian, etc.). In August 1984, the federal government opened the scheme up to include Malaysians of Portuguese descent, in effect conferring on them the status of "honorary *bumiputras.*" In addition to being of demonstrable Portuguese descent, potential applicants had to hold Malaysian citizenship, profess the Catholic faith, be able to speak Kristang, and be endorsed by the *Regedor* (*The Star,* August 4, 1984). The last two conditions were particularly significant: the language requirement was an attempt to exclude wealthy, upper-class Eurasians from Penang and Kuala Lumpur while the required endorsement gave official status to the *Regedor* of the Portuguese Settlement, effectively making him the de facto national leader of Eurasians of Portuguese descent.

10. Daus (1989, 26) suggests that Portuguese Eurasians have become a success-ful part of this tourist package because they have one thing to offer: prestige. While I agree that this is true, it is a further example of Settlement people making the most of their opportunities. If the marketing theme had been

anything other than "Historical Malacca," they would not have been able to capitalize on their past to such an extent.

11. It is interesting, too, that although publicity material always describes The Vintage as a Malaccan Portuguese group, only on rare occasions do they perform any of the songs or dances of the Settlement. (One time, when Joe Lazaroo happened to be in up Kuala Lumpur and stopped off unexpectedly to catch their lunchtime show, Basil sang "O Malhão" as a joke.) Most of the time, they sing popular American and Malay songs.

12. I am grateful to one of my anonymous readers for this final insight.

Books and Articles

Acciaioli, Greg. 1985. "Culture as Art: From Practice to Spectacle in Indonesia." *Canberra Anthropology* 8, nos. 1–2: 148–72.

Agência Geral do Ultramar. 1954. *Relação da Primeira Viagem do Ministro do Ultramar às Províncias do Oriente no Ano de MCMLII,* vol. 2. Lisbon: Agência Geral do Ultramar, Divisão de Publicações e Biblioteca.

Aggarwal, Ravina. 1996. "The Monastery and the Marketplace: Women's Power and Ethnographic 'Truth' in the Ladakh Himalayas." Paper presented at Smith College, Northampton, Mass., 22 February.

A La Bosco [Lazaroo, George Bosco]. 1968. "An Enterprise of Social Value." *The Rally* 22, no. 11 (November): 440.

A.M.F. 1935. "Our Penang Association: History of Foundation and Tribute to Founders." *The Eurasian Review* 1, no. 4 (May): 14–15.

Andaya, Barbara Watson, and Leonard Y. Andaya. 1982. *A History of Malaysia.* London: Macmillan.

Anderson, Benedict. 1983. *Imagined Communities: Reflections on the Origin and Spread of Nationalism.* New York: Verso.

Aragon, Lorraine V. 1996. "Suppressed and Revised Performances: *Raego'* Songs of Central Sulawesi." *Ethnomusicology* 40, no. 3: 413–39.

Armstrong, Lucile. 1948. *Dances of Portugal.* London: Max Parrish. Reprinted in 1950 and 1957.

Averill, Gage. 1997. *A Day for the Hunter, A Day for the Prey: Popular Music and Power in Haiti.* Chicago: University of Chicago Press.

Baxter, Alan. 1985. "Kristang (Melaka Creole Portuguese)." Ph.D. dissertation, Australian National University, Canberra.

———. 1987. "Kristang-English Dictionary." Typescript.

Bird, Isabella. 1990. *The Golden Chersonese: The Malayan Travels of a Victorian Lady.* Singapore: Oxford University Press. First published in 1883 by John Murray, London.

Boon, James. 1990. *Affinities and Extremes: Crisscrossing the Bittersweet Ethnology of East Indies History, Hindu-Balinese Culture and Indo-European Allure.* Chicago: University of Chicago Press.

Boxer, C. R. 1961. *Four Centuries of Portuguese Expansion, 1415–1825: A Succinct Survey.* Johannesburg: Witwatersrand University Press.

———. 1963. *Race Relations in the Portuguese Colonial Empire 1415–1825.* Oxford: Clarendon Press.

———. 1969. *The Portuguese Seaborne Empire 1415–1825.* London: Hutchinson.

Breckenridge, Carol A., and Peter van der Veer, eds. 1993. *Orientalism and the Postcolonial Predicament: Perspectives on South Asia.* Philadelphia: University of Pennsylvania Press.

Bruner, Edward M. 1994. "Abraham Lincoln as Authentic Reproduction: A Critique of Postmodernism." *American Anthropologist* 96, no. 2: 397–415.

———. 1995. "The Ethnographer/Tourist in Indonesia." In *International Tourism: Identity and Change,* ed. Marie-Françoise Lanfant, Edward M. Bruner, and John Allcock, 224–41. London: Sage.

———. 1996. "Tourism in the Balinese Borderzone." In *Displacement, Diaspora, and Geographies of Identity,* ed. Smadar Lavie and Ted Swedenburg, 157–79. Durham, N.C.: Duke University Press.

Bruner, Edward M., and Barbara Kirshenblatt-Gimblett. 1994. "Maasai on the Lawn: Tourist Realism in East Africa." *Cultural Anthropology* 9, no. 4: 435–70.

Cardoso, Abel, Jr. 1978. *Carmen Miranda: A Cantora do Brasil.* N.p.: Abel Cardoso.

Central Intelligence Agency. 1994. "Malaysia." In *The World Factbook* (1994 edition). http://www.odci.gov/cia/publications/factbook/my.html

Chin Yik Poh. 1967–68. "The Portuguese Settlement of Malacca." Academic Exercise, University of Singapore, Dept. of Geography.

Chopyak, James D. 1986. "Music in Modern Malaysia: A Survey of the Musics Affecting the Development of Malaysian Popular Music." *Asian Music* 18, no. 1: 111–38.

Clammer, John R. 1986. "Ethnic Processes in Urban Melaka." In *Ethnicity and Ethnic Relations in Malaysia,* ed. Raymond Lee, 47–72. DeKalb, Ill.: Center for Southeast Asian Studies, Northern Illinois University.

Clifford, James. 1997. *Routes: Travel and Translation in the Late Twentieth Century.* Cambridge, Mass.: Harvard University Press.

Cohen, Erik. 1988. "Authenticity and Commoditization in Tourism." *Annals of Tourism Research* 15: 371–86.

Comaroff, John, and Jean Comaroff. 1992. *Ethnography and the Historical Imagination.* Boulder, Colo.: Westview Press.

Cortesão, Armando. 1944. *The Suma Oriental of Tomé Pires: An Account of the East, from the Red Sea to Japan, Written in Malacca and India in 1512–1515.* London: The Hakluyt Society.

Cunningham, Clark E. 1989. "Celebrating a Toba Batak National Hero: An Indonesian Rite of Identity." In *Changing Lives, Changing Rites: Ritual and Social Dynamics in Philippine and Indonesian Uplands,* ed. Susan D. Russell and Clark E. Cunningham, 167–200. Ann Arbor: University of Michigan Press.

Daus, Ronald. 1989. *Portuguese Eurasian Communities in Southeast Asia.* Singapore: Institute of Southeast Asian Studies.

de Silva, Patrick. n.d. Untitled manuscript describing the history, customs, and traditions of Portuguese Eurasians in Melaka. Typescript.

———. 1979. "Lingo-Cultural Aspects of the Malaysian-Portuguese Community." In *Save the Portuguese Community,* 11–15. Malacca: SPCC.

———. 1987. "A Traditional Malacca Portuguese-Eurasian Engajement [*sic*] and Marriage." *Review of Culture* 3: 84–88.

———. 1990. "The Portuguese Settlement in Brief." *Festa San Pedro 1990: Souvenir Program.* Melaka: Festa San Pedro Organising Committee.

de Souza, Francisco. 1710. *O Oriente conquistado a Jesus Christo pelos Padres da Companhia de Jesus.* 2 vols. Lisbon.

Dickinson, A. H. 1941. "The History of the Creation of the Malacca Police." *Journal of the Malayan Branch of the Royal Asiatic Society* 19, no. 2: 251–83.

dos Santos Ferreira, José. 1994. Liner notes to Tuna Macaense *Macau Sã Assi.* Macau: Tradisom 007.

Eurasian Association, Penang. 1934a. "The Eurasian Volunteer Company, Malacca." *The Eurasian Review* 1, no. 2 (October): 22.

———. 1934b. "Selangor Eurasian Association: A Brief History." *The Eurasian Review* 1, no. 2 (October): 12–14.

———. 1987. *Penang Eurasian Community: Population Survey, 1987.* Penang: Penang Eurasian Association.

Eurasian Association, Singapore. 1989. *70 Years Celebration* [souvenir program from the Eurasian Association's seventieth anniversary gala ball. Hilton Hotel, 8 December]. Singapore: Singapore Eurasian Association.

Feintuch, Burt. 1993. "Musical Revival as Musical Transformation." In *Transforming Tradition: Folk Music Revivals Examined,* ed. Neil V. Rosenberg, 183–93. Urbana: University of Illinois Press.

Fernando, C. M. 1894. "The Music of Ceylon." *The Journal of the Ceylon Branch of the Royal Asiatic Society of Great Britain and Ireland* 13, no. 45: 183–189.

Handler, Richard, and Jocelyn Linnekin. 1984. "Tradition, Genuine or Spurious." *Journal of American Folklore* 97, no. 385: 273–90.

Hiebert, Murray. 1995. "A Sea Change." *Far Eastern Economic Review* 10 (August): 50–51.

Hobsbawm, Eric. 1983. "Introduction: Inventing Traditions." In *The Invention of Tradition,* ed. Eric Hobsbawn and Terrence Ranger, 1–14.

Hobsbawm, Eric, and Terrence Ranger. 1983. *The Invention of Tradition.* Cambridge: Cambridge University Press.

Howell, E. W. 1934. "Proposed Eurasian Association in Malacca." *The Eurasian Review* 1, no. 2 (October): 23–24.

Hoyt, Sarniah Hayes. 1993. *Old Malacca.* Kuala Lumpur: Oxford University Press.

Jackson, Kenneth David. 1990. *Sing without Shame: Oral Traditions in Portuguese Creole Verse.* Amsterdam: John Benjamins Publishing Company; Macau: Instituto Cultural de Macau.

———. 1998. Liner notes to *Desta Barra Fora: Damão, Diu, Cochim, Korlai.* Vol. 4 in A viagem dos sons/The journey of sounds. Vila Verde, Portugal: Tradisom VS04.

João do Rio [pseud. of Paolo Barreto]. 1909. *Fados, Canções, e Danças de Portugal.* Rio de Janeiro: H. Garnier.

Kahn, Joel S. 1992. "Class, Ethnicity and Diversity: Some Remarks on Malay Culture in Malaysia." In *Fragmented Vision: Culture and Politics in Contemporary Malaysia,* ed. Joel S. Kahn and Francis Loh Kok Wah, 158–78. North Sydney: Allen and Unwin.

Keeler, Ward. 1996. "Review of *On the Subject of 'Java,'* by John Pemberton." *The Journal of Asian Studies* 55, no. 1: 226–27.

Kessler, Clive S. 1992. "Archaism and Modernity: Contemporary Malay Political Structure." In *Fragmented Vision: Culture and Politics in Contemporary Malaysia,* ed. Joel S. Kahn and Francis Loh Kok Wah, 133–57. North Sydney: Allen and Unwin.

Kipp, Rita Smith. 1996. *Dissociated Identities: Ethnicity, Religion, and Class in an Indonesian Society.* Ann Arbor: University of Michigan Press.

Kirshenblatt-Gimblett, Barbara. 1988. "Authenticity and Authority in the Representation of Culture: The Poetics and Politics of Tourist Production." In *Kulturkontakt, Kulturkonflikt: Zur Erfahrung des Fremden. 26 Deutscher Volkskundekongress in Frankfurt vom 28 Sept. bis 2 Oktober 1987,* 59–69. Frankfurt am Main: Institut für Kulturanthropologies und Europäische Ethnologie, Universität Frankfurt am Main.

———. 1998. *Destination Culture: Tourism, Museums, and Heritage.* Berkeley and Los Angeles: University of California Press.

Knowlton, Edgar C. 1964. "Guest Language: Malaysian Portuguese (2)." *The Linguist* 26, no. 9: 239–41.

Kornhauser, Bronia. 1978. "In Defence of Kroncong." In *Studies in Modern Indonesian Music,* ed. Margaret J. Kartomi, 104–83. Monash Papers on Southeast Asia, No. 7. Clayton, Victoria: Monash University.

Lazaroo, George Bosco. ca. 1953. Program for Christmas Concert. Typescript.

———. 1956. Program for Festa di San Pedro Concert. Typescript.

Leça, Armando. ca. 1983. *Música Popular Portuguesa.* Porto: Domingos Barreira.

Luhrmann, T. M. 1996. *The Good Parsi: The Fate of a Colonial Elite in a Postcolonial Society.* Cambridge, Mass.: Harvard University Press.

MacCannell, Dean. 1973. "Staged Authenticity: On Arrangements of Social Space in Tourist Settings." *American Journal of Sociology* 79, no. 3: 589–603.

———. 1976. *The Tourist: A New Theory of the Leisure Class.* New York: Schocken.

———. 1992. "Reconstructed Ethnicity: Tourism and Cultural Identity in Third World Communities." In *Empty Meeting Grounds: The Tourist Papers,* 158–71. London: Routledge.

Maxwell, W. George. 1911. "Barretto de Resende's Account of Malacca." *Journal of the Straits Branch of the Royal Asiatic Society* 60: 1–24.

McGilvray, Dennis B. 1982. "Dutch Burghers and Portuguese Mechanics: Eurasian Ethnicity in Sri Lanka." *Comparative Studies in Society and History* 24, no. 2: 235–63.

Mohd Anis Md Nor. 1990. "The Zapin Melayu Dance of Johor: From Village to a National Performance Tradition." Ph.D. dissertation, University of Michigan.

———. 1993. *Zapin: Folk Dance of the Malay World.* Singapore: Oxford University Press.

Moura, Abel. 1994. *Cancioneiro de Música Tradicional Portuguesa: Repertório do Grupo de Danças e Cantares do Clube de Macau.* Macau: Instituto Português do Oriente.

Nash, Manning. 1989. *The Cauldron of Ethnicity in the Modern World.* Chicago: University of Chicago Press.

O'Neill, Brian Juan. 1998. "Kristang Family Heritage (Preliminary Remarks)." In *Save Our Portuguese Heritage Conference '95 Malacca, Malaysia,* ed. Gerard Fernandis, 65–74. Malacca: Gerard Fernandis.

PKKPPM (Panel Ketua Kampung Perkampungan Portugis Melaka, Portuguese Settlement *Regedor*'s Panel, Malacca). 1996. Memo concerning Festa di San Pedro Celebration on June 29, 1996. Typescript. 10 March.

Peacock, James. 1968. *Rites of Modernization: Symbols and Social Aspects of Indonesian Proletarian Drama.* Chicago: University of Chicago Press.

Pemberton, John. 1994. *On the Subject of "Java."* Ithaca, N.Y.: Cornell University Press.

Picard, Michel. 1990. "'Cultural Tourism' in Bali: Cultural Performances as Tourist Attractions." *Indonesia* 49: 37–74.

———. 1996. *Bali: Cultural Tourism and Touristic Culture.* Singapore: Archipelago Press.

Pintado, Fr. Manuel Joachim. 1974. *Survival through Human Values of Religion–Culture–Language.* Malacca: Fr. M. J. Pintado.

Portuguese Settlement Funeral Association. 1991. Statement of Account: Year Ending 2/28/91. 1 June. Typescript.

Prakash, Gyan, ed. 1995. *After Colonialism: Imperial Histories and Postcolonial Displacements.* Princeton, N.J.: Princeton University Press.

Pyrard de Laval, François. 1888. *The Voyage of François Pyrard of Laval to the East Indies, the Maldives, The Moluccas, and Brazil.* Translated by Albert Gray. 2 vols. London: The Hakluyt Society.

Quincy, Josiah, ed. 1968. *The Journals of Major Samuel Shaw, First American Consul at Canton. With a Life of the Author.* Taipei: Ch'eng-Wen Publishing Company.

Rahmah Bujang. 1975. *Sejarah Perkembangan Drama Bangsawan Di Tanah Melayu dan Singapura* [The History of the Development of *Bangsawan* Drama in Malaya and Singapore]. Kuala Lumpur: Dewan Bahasa dan Pustaka.

———. 1992. "Seni Bangsawan Baru: Pro dan Kontra" [The New Art of *Bangsawan:* Pros and Cons]. Paper presented at the international seminar "Southeast Asian Traditional Performing Arts: The State of the Art," August 10–13, 1992, Universiti Sains Malaysia, Penang. Typescript.

Robless, Aloysius E., and Aloysius Sta. Maria. n.d. "The Malaysian Portuguese: Their Customs, Traditions, Culture and Language—Kristang." Typescript.

Rosaldo, Renato. 1989. *Culture and Truth: The Remaking of Social Analysis.* Boston: Beacon Press.

Rubenstein, Carol. 1992. "The Cultural Show: Is It Culture Or What and for Whom?" *Asian Music* 23, no. 2: 1–62.

Sta. Maria, Bernard. 1979. "Evolution of Malaysian Portuguese Community." In *Save the Portuguese Community,* 6–9. Malacca: SPCC.

———. 1982. *My People, My Country: The Story of the Malacca Portuguese Community.* Malacca: The Malacca Portuguese Development Centre.

Sta. Maria, Joseph. 1987. "Letter to the Chairmen of the Selangor, Perak, Penang, and Kedah Eurasian Associations." 9 September. Typescript.

———. 1994. *Undi Nos By Di Aki?* [Where Do We Go from Here?]. Malacca: Joseph Sta. Maria.

Sta. Maria, Rachel. 1979. "The Origin of the Portuguese Settlement." In *Save the Portuguese Community,* 20–24. Malacca: SPCC.

Sarkissian, Margaret. 1987. "Armenian Musical Culture in Toronto: Political and Social Divisions in an Immigrant Community." Master's thesis, University of Illinois at Urbana-Champaign.

———. 1993. "Music, Identity, and the Impact of Tourism in the Portuguese Settlement, Melaka, Malaysia." Ph.D. dissertation, University of Illinois at Urbana-Champaign.

———. 1995–96. "'Sinhalese Girl' Meets 'Aunty Annie': Competing Expressions of Ethnic Identity in the Portuguese Settlement, Melaka, Malaysia." *Asian Music* 27, no. 1: 37–62.

——. 1997. "Cultural Chameleons: Portuguese Eurasian Strategies for Survival in Postcolonial Malaysia." *Journal of Southeast Asian Studies* 28, no. 2: 249–62.

——. 1998a. "Tradition, Tourism, and the Cultural Show: Malaysia's Diversity on Display." *Journal of Musicological Research* 17: 87–112.

——. 1998b. Liner notes to *Kantiga di Padri să Chang: Malaca*. Vol. 5 in *A viagem dos sons*/The journey of sounds. Vila Verde, Portugal: Tradisom VS 05.

——. 1999. "Patron Saints, Decorated Boats, and the Sugar Cane Story: Holidays and Holy Days in the Construction of a Malaysian Community." In *Social Allegiances and Boundaries: Essays on Southeast Asia in Honor of Clark E. Cunningham*, ed. Susan Russell and Lorraine Aragon. Tempe: Arizona State University, Center for Southeast Asian Studies.

Save the Portuguese Community Committee, Research Division. 1979. *Save the Portuguese Community*. Malacca: SPCC.

Seebass, Tilman. n.d. "Presence and Absence of Portuguese Musical Elements in Indonesia: An Essay on the Mechanics of Musical Acculturation." Duke University, Working Papers in Asian/Pacific Studies. Typescript.

Shils, Edward. 1981. *Tradition*. Chicago: University Press of Chicago.

Silva Rêgo, Padre António da. 1941. "Apontamentos para o estudo do dialecto Português de Malaca." *Boletim Geral das Colónias* 17, no. 198: 3–235.

——. 1959. *Portuguese Colonization in the Sixteenth Century: A Study of the Royal Ordinances* (Regimentos). Johannesburg: Witwatersrand University Press.

Singho, Michael. 1998. "Reclamation and the Portuguese Settlement." In *Save Our Portuguese Heritage Conference '95 Malacca, Malaysia*, ed. Gerard Fernandis, 22–30. Malacca: Gerard Fernandis.

Stier, Wayne. 1990. "Say Hello Joe." *Wings* [MAS in-flight magazine]. June issue, 35–38.

Tan Chee Beng. 1988. *The Baba of Melaka: Culture and Identity of a Chinese Peranakan Community in Malaysia*. Petaling Jaya, Selangor: Pelanduk Publications.

Tan Sooi Beng. 1984. *Ko-Tai: A New Form of Chinese Urban Street Theatre in Malaysia*. Reasearch Notes and Discussions Paper, no. 40. Singapore: Institute of Southeast Asian Studies.

——. 1988. *The "Phor Tor" Festival in Penang: Deities, Ghosts, and Chinese Ethnicity*. Working Paper, no. 51. Clayton: Center of Southeast Asian Studies, Monash University.

——. 1989a. "From Popular to 'Traditional' Theater: the Dynamics of Change in *Bangsawan* of Malaysia." *Ethnomusicology* 33, no. 2: 217–74.

————. 1989b. "A Social and Stylistic History of *Bangsawan,* ca. 1880–1980: Correspondences Between Social-Historical and Musical-Theatrical Change." Ph.D. dissertation, Monash University.

————. 1992. "Towards a Social-Historical Ethnomusicology: *Bangsawan* as a Case Study." Paper presented at the colloquium on "Music of Southeast Asia: A Workshop on Music Research in Southeast Asia," July 16–17, 1992, Universiti Kebangsaan Malaysia. Typescript.

————. 1993. *Bangsawan: A Social and Stylistic History of Popular Malay Opera.* Singapore: Oxford University Press.

————. 1996–97. "The 78 RPM Record Industry in Malaya Prior to World War II." *Asian Music* 28, no. 1: 1–41.

Texeira, Fr. Manuel. 1961. *The Portuguese Missions at Malacca and Singapore (1511–1958).* 2 vols. Lisbon: Agência Geral do Ultramar. Reprinted in 3 volumes in 1987. Macau: Instituto Cultural de Macau.

Thomas, Nicholas. 1994. *Colonialism's Culture: Anthropology, Travel and Government.* Princeton, N.J.: Princeton University Press.

Thomas, Philip L. 1986. *Like Tigers around a Piece of Meat: The Baba Style of Dondang Sayang.* Singapore: Institute of Southeast Asian Studies.

Tuna Macaense. 1994. Tuna Macaense *Macau Sã Assi.* Macau: Tradisom 007.

Turner, Victor W. 1986. "Dewey, Dilthey, and Drama: An Essay in the Anthropology of Experience." In *The Anthropology of Experience,* ed. Victor W. Turner and Edward M. Bruner, 33–44. Urbana: University of Illinois Press.

Waterman, Christopher A. 1990. "'Our Tradition is a Very Modern Tradition': Popular Music and the Construction of Pan-Yoruba Identity." *Ethnomusicology* 34, no. 3: 367–79.

Wu Hung. 1995. *Monumentality in Early Chinese Art and Architecture.* Stanford: Stanford University Press.

Young, Robert J. C. 1995. *Colonial Desire: Hybridity in Theory, Culture and Race.* London: Routledge.

Newspapers

Malacca Guardian (MG)

June 25, 1928	"The Portuguese Convent—A Successful Concert."
Apr 22, 1929	"Governor of Macao. Distinguished Official Visits Malacca."
May 9, 1932	"The Future of Malacca Eurasians."
Apr 23, 1933	"Girls' Sports Club. First Annual Report" and "Volunteers Entertain Their Commanding Officer. Brilliant Success of Amateur Show."
Oct 2, 1933	"Portuguese Settlement Malacca."
Oct 30, 1933	"Portuguese Settlement."

Oct 22, 1934	"The Eurasian Association."
Oct 29, 1934	"Agitation to Form Local Eurasian Association Takes Shape."
Nov 19, 1934	"Malacca Girls' Sports Club. Excellent Organisation."
Dec 24, 1934	"Eurasian Association Meeting."
Jan 20, 1936	Local news section: Wedding of Clement de Silva and Ida Rodrigues.
Mar 26, 1936	"Malacca Eurasian Association. 1st Annual Report."
June 29, 1936	"Malacca Fishermen's Petition."
Apr 5, 1937	"Holy Week in Malacca."
May 17, 1937	"Mirth and Merriment at Portuguese Settlement. Coronation Sports for Poor Eurasian Children."
Apr 25, 1938	"Eurasians Hold Easter Dance."
Jan 9, 1939	"Portuguese Vessel Visits Malacca After Interval of 300 Years."
Feb 19, 1940	"Plea on Behalf of Malacca Fisherfolk."

Malay Mail (MM)

Dec 6, 1968	"Portuguese Dances and Songs at K.L. Concert." By Calvin Goh.
Dec 29, 1968	"Move with the Times Call to Malacca Portuguese."
Sep 26, 1992	"The Swirling Dancers: Focus on Malacca's Attractions."

The New Straits Times (NST)

Oct 27, 1987	"Portuguese Settlement Row: CM Allays Fear."
Aug 23, 1990	"Historical Zone Gazetted by Malacca." By P. Selvarani.
Dec 19, 1990	"Feast for Country Music Fans." By Kharleez Zubin.
Aug 5, 1991	"Honouring the Legacy of the Trez Amigos." By Anne Haslam.
Sep 26, 1992	"Local Band Cries Foul." By Zieman.
Mar 10, 1993	Cartoon by Lat.

Parade [*The Sunday Star* Magazine]

Jan 4, 1976	"A Proud Race Tells of Their Hardship." By Karen Kraal.

Singapore Herald

Apr 12, 1971	"Rosil is Still Dancing at 71."

Singapore Standard (SS)

Mar 13, 1953	"Saint's Relics in Malacca." By Percy Joseph.
Mar 16, 1953	"Thousands Show Deep Faith in Saint's Relic." By Percy Joseph.
Mar 21, 1953	"Portuguese Envoy at the Centenary."

Mar 23, 1953   "Pageant on Life of St. Francis Xavier."

The Straits Times
Mar 20, 1953   "Their Old Beliefs and Ruined Castles Glow Once More in Malacca's Historic Pageant for a Saint." By Patrick Keith.
Dec 9, 1968   "Malaysians with 500 Years of History."

The Sunday Mail
Jul 3, 1977   "Casting Their Cares Aside for St. Peter." By Susan Lim.

The Star
Aug 4, 1984   "Portuguese Thank Government for ASN."
Mar 27, 1985   "A Taste of Portuguese Culture." By M. Veera Pandiyan.
Aug 20, 1987   "Portuguese Site Woes." By. M. Veera Pandiyan.
Nov 2, 1992   "Portuguese Group is Top Cultural Troupe."
Mar 3, 1994   Letter to the editor: "Malacca Seafront is Vital." By Michael G. Singho.
June 26, 1996   "Fishermen hold 'coffin' protest."

The Sun
Apr 22, 1996   Letter to the editor: "Let's Not Make the Portuguese Community Extinct." By Michael Singho.
Jul 5, 1996   "Slow Developers May Lose Projects in Malacca." By Martin Carvalho.
Jul 7, 1996   "Reclamation Work State Can Be Proud Of." By Abu Yamin Salam.

The Sunday Star
Oct 25, 1987   "But for a File. . ."
Aug 7, 1994   "Reclaiming Land in the Dutch Tradition." By A. Letchumanan and Christy Yoong.

Unidentified newspaper clipping
May 1952   "Malacca Goes Gay to Greet the Senhor from Portugal." By Roy Ferroa.

Interviews

AC: Andrew Carvalho. June 6, 1991.

ASM: Aloysius Sta. Maria. June 24, 1991.

CRK: Christine (Rodrigues) Kanagarajah. March 19, 1991.

FJS: Frederick James Scully. June 26, 1991.

GBL: George Bosco Lazaroo. June 1, 1991; June 9, 1991.

HSM: Horace Sta. Maria. July 15, 1991.

IRS: Ida (Rodrigues) de Silva. January 1, 1991.

JBL: Emmanuel "Joe" Bosco Lazaroo. June 17, July 14, 1996; August 27, 1997.

JTC: Josephine (Theseira) de Costa. July 1, 1991.

LCB: Lim Chow Beng. May 30, 1991.

MBS: Mohamad bin Saib. April 3, 1991.

NF: Noel Felix. July 17, 1990, November 14, 1990, June 30, 1991, July 5, 1991, July 18, 1996.

PDS: Patrick de Silva. October 22, 1990.

SD: Sister Dot. July 5, 1998.

SFT: Stephen Fabiano Theseira. July 3, 1991.

TM: Theodore Moissinac. July 31, 1991.

DATE DUE

			Printed in USA

HIGHSMITH #45230